*National Fire Service
Incident Management System*

Model Procedures Guide for Emergency Medical Incidents

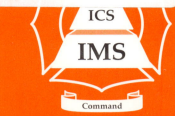

First Edition

*Prepared by the National Fire Service
Incident Management System Consortium
Model Procedures Committee*

Published by

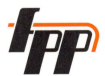

Fire Protection Publications
Oklahoma State University

*ISBN 0-87939-137-5
Library of Congress 96-61971*

Cover photo courtesy of City of Phoenix Fire Department

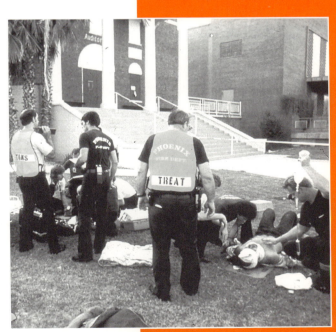

Courtesy of City of Phoenix Fire Department

RECYCLABLE

Statement of Purpose

This document is designed as a guide to assist emergency service organizations in the implementation of an Incident Management System (IMS). It may also serve as a model from which a jurisdiction may design its own plan of operation for use during emergency incidents. Once adopted by the jurisdiction and with appropriate training of personnel, it provides an easily understood organizational structure and guidelines to follow during emergency incidents.

This model encourages the use of an Incident Management System for Emergency Medical Incidents and integration for other related events and incidents. It provides guidelines for its use on routine calls as well as allowing for expansion of the organization to meet the needs of a more complex or escalating incident.

The daily use and familiarization of the concepts and guidelines of the Incident Management System model will encourage jurisdictional and statewide standardization. This will allow all emergency service providers to be better organized, improve their adaptability, and become more expedient in their operational service delivery.

Note: The original Incident Management System Model Procedures Guide for Structural Firefighting, developed by the National Fire Service Incident Management Consortium, is the basis for this document. It is intended to be used as a companion document to share the knowledge, information, and lessons learned by the members and organizations of the Consortium. It is intended for use by the fire service and related emergency service agencies to saves lives and reduce long-term disabilities of persons affected by emergency medical incidents.

Some changes have been made from the original document for editorial purposes in reference to: the basic organizational layout of the document, procedures and guidelines, and for clarification with respect to the larger group of emergency service agencies involved in responding with the Fire Service to emergency medical incidents.

Copyright @ 1996 National Fire Service Incident Management Consortium

Copyright Waiver

The National Fire Service Incident Management System Consortium grants to the user of this document permission to photocopy all or part of the procedure, as long as it is not altered nor offered for resale.

Further, the purpose of the procedure is to provide a model procedure for fire departments and other agencies to use in the design and adoption of an Incident Management System and related standard operating guidelines. Users are encouraged to use all or part of the document for that purpose.

When portions of this publication are photocopied, they should be accompanied by the following courtesy line: "Source: National Fire Service Incident Management Consortium."

Table of Contents

Foreword 1

1 Command Procedures
- A. Purpose 5
- B. Responsibilities of Command 5
- C. Functions of Command 6
- D. Establishing Command 6
- E. Command Options 8
- F. Passing Command 9
- G. Transfer of Command 10
- H. General Considerations 11
- I. Organizational Hierarchy 12

2 Command Structure
- A. Incident Management System Operations 17
- B. Command Organization 18
- C. Command Structure (Division/Group or Sector) 20
- D. Establishing Tactical Level Management Units: Basic Operational Approach 21

3 The Basic Command Organization
- A. Responding to the Emergency Medical Incident 29
- B. Expanded Organization — Reinforced Response for Emergency Medical Incidents 41
- C. Summary 47

4 Command Structure — Branches
- A. Expanding the Organization — Branches 51
- B. Branches 51
- C. Functional Branch Structure 54
- D. Branches with Operations Section Chief Supervision 56

5 Command Structure — Expanding the Organization
- A. Expanding the Organization — Sections 59
- B. Operations Section 60

    C. The Incident Commander's Role and Responsibilities After the Activation of an Operations Section Chief 61
    D. Staging Areas 62
    E. Planning Section 62
    F. Logistics Section 63
    G. Incident Command Staff 65

6 Unified Command
    A. Single Command — Incident Commander 69
    B. Unified Command 70
    C. Single/Unified Command Differences 71
    D. Unified Command — Integrating Third Service EMS Agencies 71

Appendices
    A. Glossary of Terms A1
    B. Communications B1
    C. Sample Triage Tags C1
    D. Sample Tactical Work Sheets for Emergency Medical Incidents D1
    E. Emergency Medical Incident Command Tool Box E1
    F. Credits F1

FOREWORD

National Fire Service Incident Management System Model For Emergency Medical Incidents

The purpose of the Incident Management System (IMS) is to provide for a systematic development of a complete, functional Command organization designed to allow for single or multi-agency use which increases the effectiveness of Command and improves responder safety.

This model system was developed by the National Fire Service Incident Management System Consortium. It combines command strategy and tactics with organizational procedures and is designed to be used for Emergency Medical Incidents. Much of the organizational design is applicable to other types of emergency incidents. The model reflects the merger of certain elements of the California FIRESCOPE Incident Command System and the Phoenix Fireground Command System.

The key elements of the system are:

The systematic development of a complete, functional organization with the major functions being Command, Operations, Planning, Logistics, and Finance/Administration.

Designed to allow for multi-agency adoption in federal, state, and local fire/rescue and EMS agencies. Therefore, organizational terminology used in the IMS is designed to be acceptable to all levels of government.

- Designed to be the basic, everyday operating system for all incidents within each agency. Therefore, the transition to large and/or multi-agency operations requires a minimum of adjustment for any of the agencies involved.

- The organization builds from the ground up, with the management of all major functions initially being the responsibility of one or just a few persons. Functional units are designed to handle the most important incident activities. As the incident grows in size and/or complexity, functional unit management is assigned to additional individuals in order to maintain a reasonable span of control and efficiency.

- Designed on the premise that the jurisdictional authority of the involved agencies will not be compromised. Each agency having legal responsibility within its jurisdiction is assumed to have full command authority within its jurisdiction at all times. Assisting agencies will normally function under the direction of the Incident Commander appointed by the jurisdiction within which the incident occurs.

- Multi-jurisdictional incidents will normally be managed under a Unified Command management structure involving a single Incident Command Post and a single Incident Action Plan — applicable to all agencies involved in the incident.

- The system is intended to be staffed and operated by qualified personnel from any agency, and a typical incident could involve the use of personnel from a variety of agencies, working in many different parts of the organization.

- The system expands and contracts organizationally based upon the needs of the incident. Span-of-control recommendations are followed closely; therefore, the organizational structure is never larger than required.

The Consortium recognizes the importance to the fire service of coordinating incident response with responders of other disciplines. An effective incident management system must provide an integrated multi-discipline approach. The IMS Model For Emergency Medical Incidents provides an overall structure that allows the successful integration of multiple disciplines, such as fire, medical, police, public works, and health services, at "all risk" emergency incidents.

Other response disciplines, such as nonfire service EMS agencies, police, and public works agencies, are encouraged to address their specific tactical needs within the overall Incident Management System structure. On multi-discipline incidents, experience has proven the critical necessity of integrating response agencies into one operational organization managed and supported by one structure. For this reason, the Consortium supports an integrated, multi-discipline organization over separate incident management systems for each organization.

The National Fire Service Incident Management System Consortium believes that any Incident Management System should be guideline-driven for the following reasons:

- Written guidelines reflect department policy on incident management.

- Guidelines provide a standardized approach to managing any incident.

- Guidelines provide predictable approaches to incident management.

- Guidelines should be applied routinely.

- Guidelines provide a training tool for emergency responders to reference.

- Guidelines provide a baseline for critiques and review of incidents.

- Guidelines make the Incident Commander's operations more effective.

The guidelines presented in this model reflect a procedural approach to the overall organizational structure of the Incident Management System as applied to emergency medical incidents. Those incidents may range from routine day-to-day events to the more complex and technical or to multiple and mass casualty incidents. The Consortium addresses various models of other "all risk" types of urban emergencies in other Consortium documents.

1

Command Procedures

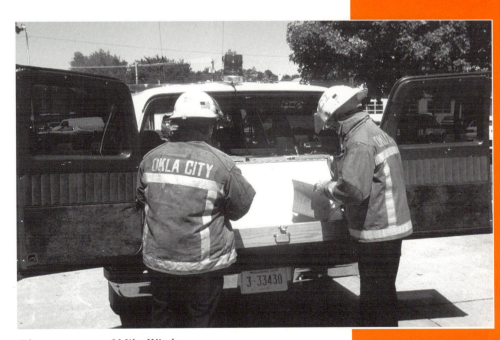

Photo courtesy of Mike Wieder

1
Command Procedures

Purpose

Fire/EMS/rescue departments respond to a wide range of emergency incidents. This model procedures guide identifies Standard Operating Guidelines (SOGs) that can be employed in establishing command for an emergency medical incident. The Incident Management System (IMS) provides for the effective management of personnel and resources and provides for their accountability, safety, and welfare. It also establishes procedures for the implementation of all IMS components required for a multiple-patient emergency medical incident.

Command Procedures are designed to:

- Fix the responsibility for command on a specific individual through a standard identification system, depending on the arrival sequence of members, companies, and chief officers.

- Ensure that a strong, direct, and visible command will be established from the onset of the incident.

- Establish an effective incident organization, defining the activities and responsibilities assigned to the Incident Commander and to other individuals operating within the Incident Management System.

- Provide a system to process information to support incident management, planning, and decision making.

- Provide a system for the orderly transfer of command to subsequent arriving officers.

Responsibilities of Command

The Incident Commander is responsible for the completion of the tactical priorities. The tactical priorities are:

1. Remove endangered persons and treat the injured.
2. Stabilize the incident and provide for life safety.
3. Ensure that the functions of extrication, triage, treatment, and transportation are established as needed and performed appropriately.
4. Conserve property and preserve evidence.

5. Provide for the safety, accountability, and welfare of all responding emergency service personnel. **This priority is ongoing throughout the incident.**

The Incident Management System is used to facilitate the completion of the tactical priorities. The Incident Commander is the person who drives the Incident Management System toward that end. The Incident Commander is responsible for building a command structure that matches the organizational needs of the incident to achieve the completion of the tactical priorities for the incident. The Functions of Command define standard activities that are performed by the Incident Commander to achieve the tactical priorities.

Functions of Command
The Functions of Command Include:

- Assume and announce Command and establish an effective operating position (Command Post).
- Rapidly evaluate the situation (size-up).
- Initiate, maintain, and control the communications process.
- Identify the overall strategy, develop an incident action plan, and assign companies and personnel consistent with plans and SOGs.
- Develop an effective Incident Management Organization.
- Provide tactical objectives.
- Review, evaluate, and revise (as needed) the action plan.
- Provide for the continuity, transfer, and termination of Command.

The Incident Commander is responsible for all of these functions. As Command is transferred, so is the responsibility for these functions. The first five (5) functions must be addressed immediately from the initial assumption of Command.

Establishing Command

The first emergency service company or member to arrive at the scene shall assume Command of the incident. The initial Incident Commander shall remain in Command until Command is transferred or the incident is stabilized and terminated.

> **Note:** Throughout this document, the term "company" represents a response unit such as an engine company, truck company, or ambulance. The term "company officer" is meant to describe the member-in-charge of that response unit. The company officer could be, for example, the captain of an engine company or the senior paramedic on an ambulance.

- The first unit or member on the scene must initiate whatever parts of the Incident Management System are needed to effectively manage the incident scene.

- A single-company incident (trash fires, single-patient E.M.S. incidents, etc.) may only require that company or unit acknowledge their arrival on the scene.

- For incidents that require the commitment of multiple companies or units, the first unit or member on the scene must establish and announce "Command," and develop an incident command structure appropriate for the incident.

The first-arriving fire department unit activates the Command process by giving an initial radio report.

The Radio Report should include:

1. Unit designation of the unit arriving on the scene.
2. A brief description of the incident situation, (i.e., building size, occupancy, haz-mat release, multi-vehicle accident, etc.).
3. Obvious conditions (working fire, haz-mat spill, multiple patients, etc.).
4. Brief description of action taken.
5. Declaration of Strategy (this applies to structure fires).
6. Any obvious safety concerns.
7. Assumption, identification, and location of Command.
8. Request or release resources as required.

   Example:

   For a single company incident —

   "Engine 5 is on the scene with a single-vehicle accident, appears minor, Engine 5 can handle."

   For a multiple company response —

   "Ladder 11 is on the scene at Parkway and 7th Street with a multi-vehicle accident, multiple patients apparent. Give me the balance of a 1st Alarm medical assignment with five ambulances. Stage additional units one block north on 7th Street. Ladder 11 will be Parkway Command."

Radio Designation:

The radio designation "Command" will be used along with the geographical location of the incident (i.e., "Parkway Command, "Metro Center Command"). This designation will not change throughout the duration of the incident. The designation of "Command" will remain with the officer currently in Command of the incident throughout the event.

Command Options

Assuming command of the incident presents several options, depending on the situation. If a chief officer, member, or unit without tactical capabilities (i.e., staff vehicle, no equipment, etc.) initiates Command, the establishment of a command post should be a top priority. At most incidents the initial Incident Commander will be a company officer.

A company officer assuming Command has a choice of modes and degrees of personal involvement in the tactical activities, but continues to be fully responsible for the Command functions. The initiative and judgment of the officer are of great importance. The modes identified are guidelines to assist the officer in planning appropriate actions. The actions initiated should conform with one of the above mentioned modes of operation.

The following command options define the company officer's direct involvement in tactical activities and the modes of command that may be utilized.

Investigation Mode:

Upon arrival, an incident may not have visible indicators of a significant emergency. These situations generally require investigation by the initial-arriving company while other units remain in a staged mode. The officer should assume Command and go with the company to investigate while utilizing a portable radio to command the incident.

Intervention Mode (Fast Attack):

Some situations demand immediate action and require the company officer's direct involvement to take an immediate action that will stabilize the incident. In these situations, the officer goes with the crew to provide the appropriate level of assistance and supervision. Examples of these situations include:

- Incident out of sight from the street (i.e., interior of building) or other scenes that are difficult to evaluate.

- Critical life safety situations (i.e., rescue, cardiac arrest, patient in burning car, etc.) which must be resolved immediately.

- Any incident where the safety and welfare of firefighters is a major concern.

- Multiple locations of patients.

Where fast intervention is critical, utilization of the portable radio will permit the officer's involvement in the initial patient care without neglecting initial command responsibilities. The Intervention mode should not last more than a few minutes and will end with one of the following:

COMMAND PROCEDURES

1. The situation is stabilized and/or adequate resources arrive on the scene.

2. The situation is not stabilized and the officer must withdraw from patient care activities and establish a command post. The company's crew remains to continue care and other support activities.

3. Command is transferred to a higher-ranking officer. When a chief officer assumes command, the chief officer may opt to return the company/unit officer to his/her crew, or assign him/her to a subordinate command support position.

Command Mode:

Certain incidents, by virtue of their obvious size, complexity, or potential for rapid expansion, require immediate strong, direct, overall command. In such cases, the company officer will initially assume an exterior, safe, and effective command position at the perimeter of the incident and maintain that position until the incident is resolved or the company officer is relieved by a higher-ranking officer. **A tactical work sheet shall be initiated and utilized to assist in managing these type of incidents (See Appendix D).**

If the company officer selects the Command Mode, the following options are available regarding the assignment of the remaining crew members:

1. The officer may "move up" within the company and place the company into action with two or more members. **One of the crew members will serve as the acting company officer and should be provided with a portable radio.** The collective and individual capabilities and experience of the crew will determine the viability of this option.

2. The officer may assign the crew members to work under the supervision of another company officer. In such cases, the officer assuming command must communicate with the officer of the other company and indicate the assignment of those personnel.

3. The officer may elect to assign the crew members to perform staff functions to assist Command.

Passing Command

In certain situations, it may be advantageous for a first-arriving officer to pass Command to the next company on the scene. This is indicated when the initial commitment of the first-arriving company requires a full crew (i.e., an immediate rescue situation) and another company is on the scene.

"Passing command" to a company that is not on the scene creates a gap in the Command process and compromises incident management. **To prevent this "gap," command shall not be passed to an officer who is not on the scene.** It is preferable to have the initial-arriving company officer continue to operate in the Intervention mode, using a portable radio, until Command can be passed to an on-scene unit.

When a chief officer arrives at the scene at the same time as the initial-arriving company, the chief officer should assume Command of the incident. Should a situation occur where a later-arriving company or chief officer cannot locate or communicate with Command (after several radio attempts), they will assume and announce their assumption of Command, and initiate whatever actions are necessary to confirm the safety and location of the missing crew.

Transfer of Command

Command is transferred to improve the quality of the Command organization. The following guidelines outline the transfer of command process. The transfer of Command through various ranking officers must be predetermined by the local departments. The following are examples of transfer procedures:

1. The first emergency service member arriving on the scene will automatically assume Command. This will normally be a company officer, but it could be any member up to and including the fire/EMS/rescue chief.

2. The first-arriving company officer will assume Command after the transfer of command procedures have been completed (assuming an equal or higher-ranking officer has not already assumed Command).

3. The first-arriving chief officer should assume Command of the incident following transfer of command procedures.

4. The second-arriving chief officer should report to the command post for assignment.

5. Later-arriving, higher-ranking chief officers may choose to assume Command, or assume advisor positions.

6. Assumption of Command is discretionary for senior level officers. This does not release them of responsibility and accountability for incident actions.

Within the chain of command, the actual transfer of command will be regulated by the following procedures:

1. The officer assuming Command will communicate by radio or face-to-face with the person being relieved. Face-to-face is the preferred method to transfer Command.

2. The person being relieved will brief the officer assuming Command, indicating at least the following:
   A. Incident conditions (stable or unstable, patient locations and priorities, number of patients, hazards, etc.).
   B. Action plan for the incident.
   C. Progress toward completion of the tactical objectives.
   D. Safety considerations.
   E. Deployment and assignment of operating companies and personnel.
   F. Appraisal of need for additional resources.
3. The person being relieved of Command should review the tactical work sheet with the officer assuming Command. This sheet provides the most effective framework for Command transfer because it outlines the location and status of personnel and resources in a standard form that should be well known to all members.

The person being relieved of Command will be reassigned — based on the needs of the incident — by the officer assuming Command.

Most often, the first transfer of command takes place via radio. This occurs when a company officer is in Command and the first chief arrives on the scene and initiates the transfer of command. Only a few companies may be committed, and a radio transfer is effective. Later-arriving, higher-ranking chief officers desiring to assume Command must conduct the transfer face-to-face at the command post.

General Considerations

The response and arrival of additional ranking officers on the incident scene strengthens the overall Command function. As the incident escalates, the Incident Commander should use these officers as needed.

An emergency service organization's communications procedures should include communications necessary to gather and analyze information to plan, issue orders, and supervise operations. Radio codes (i.e. 10-codes) must be avoided in favor of "clear text," using noncoded English language.

For example:
- Assignment completed.
- Additional resources required.
- Unable to complete.
- Special information.

Note: Anyone can effect a change in tactical incident operations (in extreme situations compromising responder safety) by initiating corrective action and notifying Command of actions taken and the outcome.

The arrival of a ranking officer on the incident scene **does not** mean that Command has been automatically transferred to that officer. Command is only transferred when the outlined transfer of command process has been completed. Chief officers and staff personnel should report directly to a designated location for assignment by the Incident Commander (i.e. staging, command post, etc.).

The Incident Commander has the overall responsibility for managing an incident. Simply stated, the Incident Commander has complete authority and responsibility for the incident until properly relieved. If a higher-ranking officer wants to effect a change in the management of an incident, he/she must first be on the scene of the incident, then utilize the transfer of command procedure.

Organizational Hierarchy

The IMS organizational structure develops in a modular fashion based upon the kind, complexity, and size of an incident. The organization's staff builds from the top down with responsibility and performance placed initially with the Incident Commander. As the need exists, four separate Sections can be developed, each with several Units that may be established. The specific organizational structure established for any given incident will be based upon the management needs of the incident. If one individual can simultaneously manage all major functional areas, no further organization is required. If one or more of the areas requires independent management, an individual is named to be responsible for that area.

To understand the terms and titles used in this model procedures guide, an organizational hierarchy of command titles is provided for ease of reference and understanding.

- **Command**
- **Officer**
- **Section Chief**
- **Director**
- **Supervisor**
- **Unit Leader**
- **Manager**
- **Single Resource**

Command: Title that refers to the Incident Commander.

Officer: Title that refers to a member of the Command Staff (Information Officer, Safety Officer, Liaison Officer).

Section Chief: Title that refers to a member of the General Staff (Planning Section Chief, Operations Section Chief, Finance/Administration Section Chief, Logistics Section Chief).

Director: Title that refers to the position of Branch Director, which is in the Operations Section or Logistics Section between the tactical level management units and the Operations Section Chief (Air Operations Branch Director, Service Branch Director).

Supervisor: Title that refers to the tactical level management unit supervisors (Division/Group or Sector), which is in the Operations Section and lies between the Branch Director and Strike Team/Task Force Leader.

Unit Leader: Title that refers to a position with supervision and management responsibility of either a group of resources or a unit, such as Triage, Treatment, Transportation, Supply, etc.

Manager: Title that refers to the lowest level of supervision within the incident management system and reports to a unit leader. The only exception to this is the Staging Area Manager who reports directly to the Operations Section Chief.

Single Resource: An engine company or truck company with a company officer and crew or an ambulance with a crew.

2

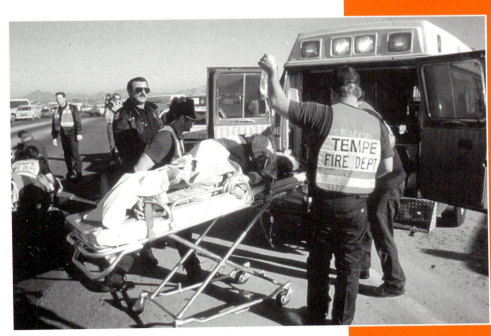

Photo courtesy of City of Phoenix Fire Department

Command Structure

2

Command Structure

It will be the responsibility of the Incident Commander to develop an organizational structure utilizing standard operating guidelines (SOGs) as soon as possible after arrival. It will also be the IC's responsibility to implement initial tactical control measures. The size and complexity of the organizational structure, obviously, will be determined by the scope of the emergency.

Incident Management System Operations

The Incident Management System (IMS) should be considered the basic incident management system to be used on any size or kind of incident. The system may be readily expanded to meet the increased needs that occur when the initial or reinforced response is determined to be inadequate by the IC.

IMS Organizational Development

The following examples are guides in using the basic Incident Management System Organization for various size incidents.

Initial Response	1-5 Increments/1st Alarm
Reinforced Response	Greater Alarm/Mutual Aid

Initial Response

The first-arriving unit or officer will assume Command until arrival of a higher-ranking officer. Upon arrival of a higher-ranking officer, he/she will be briefed by the on-scene Incident Commander. The higher-ranking officer will then assume Command.

Reinforced Response

A reinforced response will be initiated when the on-scene Incident Commander determines that the initial-response resources will be insufficient to deal with the size or complexity of the incident.

The reinforced response should be adequate to manage the needs of the incident action plan. Additional resources should be requested in a standardized, grouped response that is predicable. Piecemealing of additional resources should be avoided. Requesting a specific resource for a specific tactical assignment is not considered piecemealing.

Command Organization

The command organization must develop at a pace which stays ahead of the tactical deployment of personnel and resources. In order for the Incident Commander to manage the incident, the IC must first be able to direct, control, and track the position and function of all operating companies. Building a command organization is the best support mechanism the IC can utilize to achieve the harmonious balance between managing personnel and incident needs. Simply put, this means:

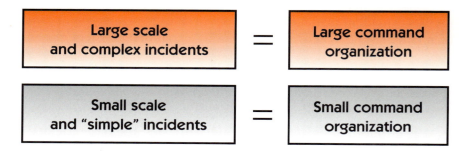

Note: The Incident Commander should always have more people working than commanding.

The basic configuration of Command includes three levels:

Strategic level: overall direction of the incident

Tactical level: assigns operational objectives

Task level: specific tasks assigned to companies

COMMAND STRUCTURE

Strategic Level:

The strategic level involves the overall Command of the incident. The Incident Commander is responsible for the strategic level of the command structure. The action plan should cover all strategic responsibilities, all tactical objectives, and all support activities needed during the entire operational period. The action plan defines where and when resources will be assigned to the incident to control the situation. This plan is the basis for developing a command organization, assigning all resources, and establishing tactical objectives.

The strategic level responsibilities include:

- Determine the appropriate strategy.
- Establish overall incident objectives.
- Set priorities.
- Develop an action plan.
- Obtain and assign resources.
- Planning — based on evaluating interventions and predicting outcomes.
- Assign specific objectives to tactical level units.

Tactical Level:

The tactical level directs operational activities toward specific objectives. Tactical level officers include Branch Directors and Division, Group, or Sector Supervisors who are in charge of grouped resources. Tactical level directors and supervisors are responsible for specific geographic areas or functions and supervising assigned personnel. A tactical level assignment comes with the authority to make decisions and assignments within the boundaries of the overall plan and safety conditions. The accumulated achievements of tactical objectives should accomplish the strategy of the action plan.

Task Level:

The task level refers to those activities normally accomplished by individual companies or specific personnel. The task level is where the work is actually done. Task level activities are routinely supervised by company officers, based on tactical objectives. The accumulated achievements of task level activities should accomplish tactical objectives.

Examples:

The most basic command structure combines all three levels of the command structure. The company officer responding on a single resource to a routine single-patient incident determines the strategy and tactics and supervises the crew doing the task.

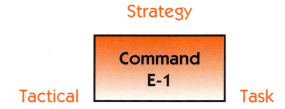

The basic structure for a "routine" incident, involving a small number of companies, requires the three levels of the command structure to be divided. The role of Command combines the strategic and tactical levels. Companies and crews report directly to Command and operate at the task level.

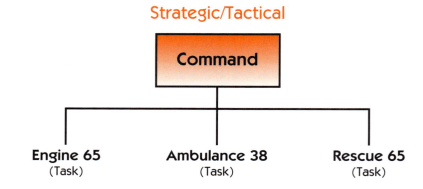

Command Structure
(Division/Group or Sector)

The terms **Divisions**, **Groups**, or **Sectors** are tactical level management units that group companies and/or resources. Divisions represent geographic operations, and groups represent functional operations. The term sector is generic and can be used for both geographic and functional operations. Since all three terms are in common use throughout the country, the local jurisdiction should select the term or terms it prefers. The following examples illustrate the use of these terms.

> **Note:** For the purpose of clarification in this document, the term "tactical level management unit" will be used when referencing a division, group, or sector.

It's important not to be too concerned about which term a local jurisdiction may prefer. What is of greater importance is the title attached to the "front end" of a tactical level position. For example, the title "Medical" clearly defines the tactical level Supervisor's responsibilities and is easily remembered and understood by all emergency service personnel working at the incident.

Establishing Tactical Level Management Units: Basic Operational Approach

The initial response of resources to a major emergency medical incident will normally require more tasks to be accomplished than there are emergency service personnel until additional resources arrive on the scene. The tendency is to treat patients, and wait well into the rescue operation before implementing the Incident Management System. This is a major error, resulting in confusion and loss of a well-coordinated and directed rescue effort. The system must be implemented with the first companies on the scene.

Complex emergency situations often exceed the capability of one officer to effectively manage the entire operation. The incident must be divided up into organizational subcomponents of certain geographic areas or functions related to the incident. This is done through the use of Divisions, Groups, or Sectors which are tactical level management units.

The use of tactical level management units in the Command organization provides a standard system for dividing the incident scene. Creating subordinate management units reduces the span of control to more manageable, smaller-sized units. This allows the Incident Commander to communicate principally with these organizational levels, rather than multiple, individual company officers. This system provides an effective command structure and incident scene organization.

Generally, tactical level management unit responsibilities should be assigned early in the incident — **typically to the first company assigned to a geographic area or function**. This early establishment of tactical level management units provides an effective incident management organization framework on which the operation can be built and expanded.

The number of tactical level management units that can be effectively managed by the Incident Commander varies. Normal span of control is three to seven. In fast-moving, complex, multiple-patient operations, a span of control of no more than five tactical level management units is indicated. In slower-moving, less-complex operations (building collapse with labor intense rescue and extrication operations), the Incident Commander may effectively manage more tactical level management units.

Where the number of tactical level management units exceeds the span of control that the Incident Commander can effectively manage, the incident organization can be expanded to meet incident needs by assigning an Operations Section Chief. The Operations Section is responsible for implementing branches and tactical level management units. Each branch is responsible for several tactical level management units and should be assigned a separate radio channel if available (see Branches).

Tactical level management unit procedures provide an array of major functions which may be selectively implemented according to the needs of a particular situation. This places responsibility for the details and execution of each particular function on a tactical level management unit supervisor.

When effective tactical elements have been established, the Incident Commander can concentrate on overall strategy and resource assignment, allowing the supervisors to manage their assigned units. The Incident Commander determines strategy and assigns tactical objectives and resources to the tactical level management units. In order to complete the tactical objectives assigned by the Incident Commander, each supervisor is responsible for the tactical deployment of the resources at his/her disposal. The tactical level management unit supervisors are also responsible for communicating needs and progress reports to Command.

Establishment of tactical level management units is primarily for the safety and accountability of personnel and to reduce the overall amount of radio communications. The tactical level management unit supervisors must constantly monitor all hazardous situations and risks to personnel, and take appropriate action to ensure that companies are operating in a safe and effective manner.

Most routine communications within the unit should be conducted in a face-to-face manner between company officers and their tactical level management unit supervisor. This process reduces unnecessary radio traffic, increases the ability to transmit critical radio communications, and allows for effective command, control, and function of assigned companies and resources.

The Incident Commander should begin to assign tactical level management units based on the following factors:

- When situations will eventually involve a number of companies or functions beyond the capability of Command to directly control, Command should initially assign tactical management responsibilities to the first companies assigned to a geographic area or function until chief officers are available.

- When Command can no longer effectively cope with (or manage) the number of companies/units currently involved in the operation.

- When companies/units are involved in complex operations (large interior or geographic area, hazardous materials, technical rescues, etc.).

- When companies/units are operating from tactical positions that Command has little or no direct control over (i.e., out of sight).

- When the situation presents special hazards and close control is required over operating companies (i.e., unstable structural conditions, hazardous materials, patient trapped in burning car).

When establishing a Division/Group or Sector position, the Incident Commander will assign each tactical level supervisor:

1. Tactical objectives.
2. A radio designation (Division/Sector, Rescue Group, Medical Group, Treatment Group, Division).
3. The identity of resources assigned to the tactical unit.

Tactical level management units will be regulated by the following guidelines:

- It will be the ongoing responsibility of Command to assign tactical level management units as required for effective emergency operations; this assignment will relate to both geographic and functional units.

- Command shall advise each tactical level management unit supervisor of specific tactical objectives. The overall strategy and plan should be provided (time permitting) so that the tactical level management unit supervisor has some idea of what's going on and how his/her assignment fits into the overall strategic plan.

- The number of companies assigned will depend upon conditions within that tactical unit. Command will maintain an awareness of the number of companies operating within a tactical level management unit and the capability of that tactical level management unit supervisor to effectively direct operations. If the supervisor cannot control the resources within the unit, he/she should notify the Incident Commander so that the assigned responsibilities can be split or other corrective action taken. In most cases, three to seven companies represent the maximum span of control for a tactical level management unit supervisor.

- The incident scene should be subdivided in a manner that makes sense. This can be accomplished by assigning Divisions to geographic locations and assigning functional responsibilities to Groups (the term Sector for either geographic or functional responsibilities may be used as predetermined by the jurisdiction having authority). Radio designation in radio communications will use the title of the unit's function or location.

- Tactical level management units will be commanded by chief officers, company officers, or any other qualified person designated by Command.

- The guideline established for general span of control is three to seven resources. However, five is typically the number at which tactical level management unit supervision by the Incident Commander should stop. The need for further tactical elements should indicate a need to develop the "Section" level of Command (see Chapters 4 and 5). This applies to operational tactical level management units. Many of the functional responsibilities, such as Information Officer, Safety, or Liaison, are preassigned to certain individuals and are driven by SOGs. These types of functional responsibilities should operate automatically and should not be included in the Incident Commander's span of control.

- Standard transfer of command procedures will be followed in transferring tactical level management unit responsibility.

- In some cases, a tactical level management supervisor may be assigned to an area/function initially to evaluate and report conditions and advise Command of needed tasks and resources. The assigned supervisor will proceed to the tactical operational area, evaluate and report conditions to the Incident Commander, and assume responsibility for directing resources and operations within his/her assigned area of responsibility.

- The supervisor must be in a position to directly supervise and monitor operations. This will require the supervisor to be equipped with the appropriate protective clothing and equipment for his/her area of responsibility. Each supervisor must be equipped with a portable communications device, and if assigned to operate within a hazard zone, must be accompanied by an additional responder.

Supervisors will be responsible for and in control of all assigned functions within their tactical level unit. This requires each supervisor to:

A. Complete objectives assigned by Command.

B. Account for all assigned personnel.

C. Ensure that operations are conducted safely.

D. Monitor work progress.

E. Redirect activities as necessary.

F. Coordinate actions with related activities and adjacent tactical level management units.

G. Monitor welfare of assigned personnel.

H. Request additional resources as needed.

I. Provide Command with essential and frequent progress reports.

J. Reallocate and release resources within the unit as appropriate.

   Note: The supervisor should be readily identifiable and maintain a visible position as much as possible. The wearing of position identification vests is very effective.

The primary function of company officers working within a tactical level management unit is to direct the operations of their individual crews in performing assigned tasks. Company officers will advise their supervisor of work progress, preferably face to face. All requests for additional resources or assistance within a tactical level management unit must be directed to the supervisor. The supervisor will communicate with next higher level of supervision," and direct requests for additional resources to Command. Command will be responsible for obtaining those resources and prioritizing their commitment.

Each supervisor will keep Command informed of conditions and progress through regular progress reports. The supervisor must limit progress reports to essential information only. Command must be advised immediately of significant changes, particularly those involving the ability or inability to complete an objective, hazardous conditions, accidents, or structural collapse.

The supervisor should avoid becoming involved in physical "task" activities (i.e., litter bearer or holding an IV). Doing so compromises the supervisor's ability to manage and control activities. This would be acceptable only in the earliest stages of the incident, with few resources on scene. As additional resources arrive, the supervisor must resume the function of a supervising role and position.

When a company is assigned from Staging to an operating tactical level management unit, the company will be told what tactical level management unit they will be reporting to and the name of the supervisor. The tactical level management unit supervisor will be informed of which particular companies or units have been assigned by the Incident Commander. It is then the responsibility of these supervisors to contact the assigned company to transmit any instructions relative to the specific action requested.

Supervisors will monitor the condition of the crews operating in their area of responsibility. Relief crews will be requested in a manner to ensure the safety of personnel and maintain progress toward the tactical unit's objectives. Supervisors will ensure an orderly reassignment of crews to Responder Rehab. Crews must report intact to the Responder Rehab in order to facilitate accountability.

Support items for all tactical level management unit supervisors include clipboards, paper, tactical work sheets (see Appendix D), radios, lights, identification vests, and personal protective gear and SCBA as needed. Any person assigned a tactical level management position should wear a vest or other markings that easily identifies his/her area of responsibility or function.

3
The Basic Command Organization

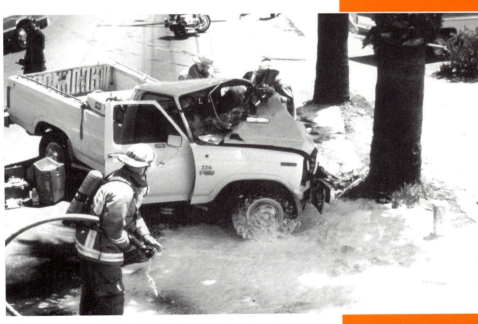
Photo courtesy of City of Phoenix Fire Department

3
The Basic Command Organization

Responding to the Emergency Medical Incident

The Incident Management System must be initiated by the first-arriving resource. IMS allows the Incident Commander to escalate and expand the command organization as needed. It begins at ground level and escalates up. Only the positions needed should be implemented, based on the number of tasks to be performed or availability of additional resources.

For example, the Incident Commander may have a structure fire with two or three smoke inhalation patients. The IC may choose to assign one company to provide all necessary medical care, and ensure that all patients are triaged, treated, and transported as needed; other companies are assigned firefighting tasks. This does not eliminate the requirement of the IC to ensure that all the functions and responsibilities are complete for any incident.

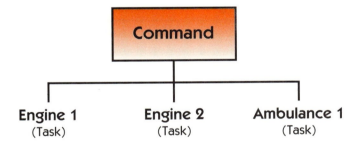

The incident management organization expands and contracts as the demands of the incident dictates.

The first-arriving company will be faced with many decisions that must be made and tasks that must be completed at any emergency medical incident. The responsibilities of the first-arriving company will include the functions of Command. The initial Incident Commander must also develop an action plan that takes into account the emergency medical care aspects of the incident and provide for:

- SAFETY hazard assessment (existing or potential) and/or life-threatening situations.

- SURVEY the scene to approximate the number and severity of patients.
- SEND information to dispatch, request additional resources as needed, and establish Command.
- SET UP the scene for emergency medical functions.
- START simple triage and rapid treatment of patients.

All major emergency medical incidents usually have one thing in common: there will likely be more tasks than responders until additional resources arrive on the scene. The tendency is to treat patients, and wait until well into the incident operations to implement an Incident Management System. This is a major error, resulting in confusion and the loss of a coordinated, directed rescue effort. The Incident Management System must be implemented with the first-arriving resources on the scene.

After initiating the incident action plan, an evaluation regarding the need for extrication is made. In many incidents, simple extrication by a few personnel is all that is needed. This allows most resources to be directed to triage, treatment, transportation of the patients, and the termination of the incident. A basic command structure with an extrication component is illustrated below.

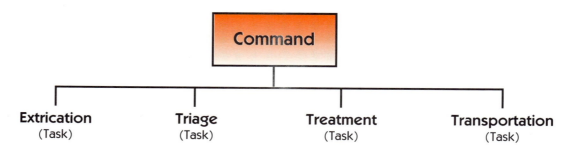

In the above diagram, the task level refers to those activities normally accomplished by individual companies or specific personnel. The task level is where the work is actually done. Task level activities are routinely supervised by company officers, based on tactical objectives. The accumulated achievements of the task level activities should accomplish tactical objectives.

The basic structure combines all three levels of the command structure. The company officer on a single-resource response determines the strategy and tactics and supervises the crew doing the task. The basic structure for a "routine" incident involving a small number of companies still requires three levels of the command structure, but the duties are combined to two positions of supervision. The role of Command combines the strategic and tactical levels while the assigned company officers report directly to Command and operate at the task level.

When the size, scope, and complexity of the incident indicates the need for a reinforced response, assignment of specific tactical level management unit supervisors and expansion of the Incident Management System is imperative. The IMS groups resources into common management units to maximize organizational effectiveness. A logical organizational grouping for emergency medical incidents includes: triage, treatment, and transport tasks and may include extrication tasks as needed. This grouping forms natural organizational positions in the Incident Management System. Additional supporting positions may be added as the incident escalates.

A general rule with any large-scale emergency medical incident is that resource commitments follow the patient flow. An initial heavy commitment of resources to the extrication and triage function may be required. At this time, the Incident Commander may deem it necessary to establish an Extrication Unit to manage the removal of all patients from the endangered area to a triage or treatment area. As patients begin to move to the treatment area, the treatment function will need to be staffed. As the demands within a tactical level management unit decrease or are no longer needed Command should be advised so that resources and personnel can be reassigned or released as needed.

Extrication Function

One of the first tactical considerations in a multiple-patient incident is the function of extrication. Extrication is utilized in incidents that require the physical disentanglement and removal of trapped patients. The Extrication Unit is responsible for locating, removing, and delivering patients to an appropriate casualty collection point, triage area, and/or treatment area. *The responsibilities of the Extrication Unit also include any initial patient treatment that may be necessary prior to disentanglement.*

The evaluation of the number of trapped patients and the complexity of their entrapment is an immediate priority. The Incident Commander will need to appoint a person to the position of Extrication Unit Leader. The Extrication Unit Leader should assign personnel to assist in the size-up if necessary.

The Extrication Unit Leader should be positioned in a readily visible location that is accessible to arriving resources and that allows a view of the extrication operation. Face-to-face communications should be used by all crews within the unit. Any person assigned a tactical level management position should wear a vest that easily identifies his/her area of responsibility or function.

Companies and crews assigned to the Extrication Unit work for and communicate with the Extrication Unit Leader. Requests for resources and progress reports must go the Extrication Unit

Leader (preferably via face to face). The Extrication Unit Leader communicates resource needs and progress reports to the next higher level of supervision established.

The Extrication Unit Leader is responsible for all patients within the extrication area until they are delivered to a designated area for further treatment and processing. Ambulatory patients with apparent minor injuries should be removed from the area or scene to a designated area as soon as possible to reduce confusion. One or more companies will be required to complete this task. These patients will eventually require assessment to determine if more serious injuries are present.

If patients are spread over a large area, companies should be assigned to a specific area or group of patients. The company assigned will have to determine the immediate needs of those patients, and provide the Extrication Unit Leader with a request for resources.

As a general rule, in order to more effectively move patients to a treatment area, all patients should be triaged and tagged first. Critical patients should be moved first, followed by delayed patients. Some situations, such as those that pose a serious safety hazard, may require that patients be moved rapidly.

When a Triage Unit is operating in the extrication area, close coordination between the Extrication and Triage Unit Leaders must take place. When triage cannot be performed in the extrication area for safety or other reasons, the Triage Unit should be placed at the exit point(s) of the extrication area. If the treatment area is close to the extrication area, triage may be performed at the entrance to the treatment area as well. If patients are in various locations, with multiple routes and exit points, then a choke point needs to be established to coordinate all personnel and patients leaving the extrication area. This configuration is commonly called a casualty collection point.

In some cases, such as confined entrapment, removing less seriously injured patients may be required in order to extricate the critical patients. These less injured patients may need to be delivered to the treatment area ahead of critical patients.

All nonambulatory patients should be moved on some type of patient transport device with cervical spine immobilization precautions taken if needed. Companies may be assigned as "litter bearers" to assist in patient movement. Pickup trucks, baggage carts, ambulance gurneys, or other similar conveyances may also be employed.

The Extrication Unit Leader must closely monitor the litter bearer operation as it is very labor intensive. Crews that are becoming exhausted should be relieved for rehabilitation or cycled to other less exhausting functions.

Advanced life support (ALS) personnel are normally not assigned to the Extrication Unit. They are better utilized in the treatment area. However, some ALS personnel may be needed in the extrication area to provide appropriate emergency medical care to patients undergoing extended/delayed extrication efforts. ALS personnel assigned to this area will be supervised by the Extrication Unit Leader.

Where patients require forcible extrication, ladder companies or other heavy rescue companies should be assigned to the Extrication Unit. These apparatus should be brought in close to the scene without blocking access to the area. If the extrication process requires specialized equipment, such as cranes or other heavy equipment, the request for these resources should be made by the Extrication Unit Leader to the next higher level of supervision.

The Extrication Unit Leader is responsible for providing site safety. This may require the commitment of personnel to staff charged hoselines, shoring, or otherwise stabilize the wreckage. If fire is involved, close coordination with firefighting tactical level management units will be required. **The safety of patients and rescue personnel must be a priority concern.**

If the incident site involves multiple extrication locations, it may be necessary to create more than one Extrication Unit. Each should be assigned a geographic designation to identify the location (i.e., North Extrication). Tactical level management unit operations may be necessary to coordinate this effort.

The Extrication Unit's responsibilities can be summarized as follows:

- Determine the location, number, and condition of all patients.
- Determine if triage is to be conducted in the extrication area, at a designated casualty collection point, or in the treatment area.
- Provide site safety for all patients and rescuers.
- Evaluate the resources needed for the extrication of trapped patients and the delivery of patients to designated medical care areas.
- Communicate resource requirements to Command.
- Allocate assigned resources appropriately.
- Supervise assigned resources.
- Extricate and deliver patients to the treatment area.
- Give frequent and timely progress reports to Command.
- Coordinate activities with other operating units as needed.
- Report to Command when all patients have been moved to the designated treatment areas.

- Maintain incident documentation as needed.
- Terminate extrication activities and reallocate assigned resources as directed by next higher level of supervision.

Triage Function

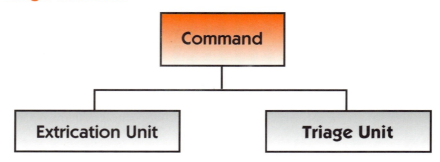

The process of quick and effective sorting of the sick and injured is a demanding endeavor and one that needs on-scene adaptive solutions. By establishing standard procedures to evaluate and treat patients, much confusion and disorder can be avoided or at least abated very quickly. The function of triage is to ensure that all persons and patients are accounted for, life-threatening injuries are assessed, and life-saving treatment is provided to stabilize patients until additional treatment resources arrive on scene. Personnel assigned to the function of triage must have basic medical knowledge and skills to conduct triage and make appropriate triage decisions.

Initial responsibility for triage at major incidents takes place in the extrication area. If the scene is safe, triage should be conducted in the impact area by appointed Triage Unit personnel. Coordination between the Extrication and Triage Unit Leaders will be required.

If safety concerns or other factors do not permit triage in the extrication/impact area, then it should be conducted at a designated casualty collection point. That point may be the entrance to the treatment area, and coordination will be required with the Treatment Unit.

When the situation dictates, the Incident Commander should appoint a Triage Unit Leader to supervise assigned personnel. The Triage Unit Leader must be in a readily visible position to oversee the triage process and to supervise the triage teams/crews, litter bearers (porter teams), and other support positions as needed, such as a temporary Morgue Manager.

The Triage Unit Leader's responsibilities can be summarized as follows:

- Determine, with close coordination with other Unit Leaders, whether triage will be conducted in the extrication area, designated casualty collection points, or at the treatment area.

- Supervise assigned triage teams and crews, litter bearers, and resources.
- Ensure that triage of patients is based upon patient conditions, that quick life-saving emergency care is provided as needed, and that patients are accounted for and tagged appropriately.
- Determine resources required for triage.
- Communicate resource requirements to Command.
- Provide frequent progress reports to Command.
- Ensure safety of all personnel assigned.
- Establish management for fatalities; designate morgue area as needed.
- Coordinate activities with other operating units and groups as needed.
- Give frequent and timely progress reports to Command.
- Report to the next level of command when all patients have been moved to the designated treatment areas and a final count of patients triaged is made.
- Maintain incident documentation as needed.
- Terminate triage activities and reallocate assigned resources as directed by next level of command.

The number of personnel needed for a Triage Unit will vary depending on the total number of patients. The following are considered to be minimum staffing needs for an initial Triage Unit development.

1 Unit Leader per triage area

1 Morgue Manager as needed

1 triage team (2 personnel) per 10 patients

1 company per 5 patients (reference to extrication/support functions)

Treatment Function

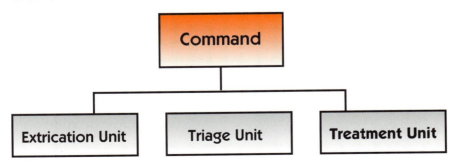

The establishment of a specific area to provide medical treatment during an emergency medical incident is dependent on the resources committed to the incident operations. The function of the Treatment Unit is to provide patient stabilization and continuing care of patients until they can be transported to a medical facility.

If enough ambulances and staff for all the patients are on scene, then the treatment area for each patient may well be at or in the ambulances. When limited resources are available on scene, a treatment area must be established to provide the necessary patient reassessment and stabilization until the patients can be transported from the scene. Of all the tactical level management units involved in a multiple-casualty incident, the operational demands and support to the Treatment Unit typically requires the heaviest commitment of personnel.

The Treatment Unit Leader is appointed by the next higher level of supervision to establish a site to manage the treatment of multiple critical and seriously injured patients. The Treatment Unit Leader is responsible for establishing a treatment area in a suitable and safe location. The treatment area must be easily accessible for patient entry and for exit to the transportation area.

The treatment area should be large enough to handle all of the patients as well as the Treatment Unit personnel — THINK BIG !

The treatment area should be established and prepared prior to the arrival of the first patient from Extrication or Triage Units. When the scene situation does not allow medical care to be provided in the area where the patients are found, the Treatment Unit Leader will advise the next level of command of the location of the specific treatment area and when the area is ready to receive patients.

The treatment area should be readily identifiable and have a visible entrance. Traffic cones or other markers should be used to make the entrance obvious, and the location should be announced to all personnel on the scene.

Personnel should be assigned to the meet and direct arriving patients to either the "immediate care" area, the "delayed care" noncritical area, or the assembly area for the walking wounded/uninjured.

The Treatment Unit is responsible for providing definitive advanced and basic life support stabilization (ALS and BLS) and continuing care of patients until they can be transported. The Treatment Unit will determine priorities for patients to be transported to medical facilities and will coordinate transportation with the Transportation Unit Leader.

Nontriaged patients arriving at the treatment area must be triaged at the entrance to the treatment area and tagged. A reassessment and tagging team must be located at the entrance for this purpose.

First-arriving patients should be placed near the exit point to the transportation area. Personnel should fill the treatment area from the exit area toward the entrance as patients are delivered. This will eliminate personnel from having to step over or around patients as they are delivered or transported.

All patients should be placed in an orderly manner in the treatment area. Adequate space must be provided between the patients to allow working room for treatment personnel. Two subareas must be established within the treatment area: an immediate care area and a delayed care area.

Most of the patients located in the "immediate care" area will require ALS treatment. Patients in the "delayed care" area may require some ALS attention, but much of their care can be delivered by BLS providers. All patients in the ambulatory/assembly area must be assessed and monitored for potential injuries by any available personnel. When adequate resources are available, all patients will be provided emergency care as indicated by injury/patient need.

Treatment personnel must perform ongoing assessment of all the patients for changes in conditions to maintain appropriate triage classification and to establish treatment and transportation priorities. The Treatment Unit Leader should assign specific personnel to monitor all patients, and provide a complete assessment of vital signs for each patient on a timed basis.

As treatment teams reassess patients and note significant patient changes (better or worse), it may be necessary to transfer some patients to a higher- or lower-priority treatment area. The patient-moving process may be very simple or complex based on the situation and location of the medical care areas. The Treatment Unit Leader should establish a process, and provide personnel to move patients quickly from one area to another.

Firefighters, paramedics, medical staff, and others may be assigned to the Treatment Unit. The Treatment Unit Leader must have specific assignments for these personnel. Additional personnel may be needed to manage the medical care areas. Support services personnel may also be needed to manage information and resource requests. Any nonfire/rescue agency personnel should be closely supervised to provide for their safety and to ensure effective operations.

The Treatment Unit Leader's responsibilities can be summarized as follows:

- Locate a LARGE, suitable treatment area and report the location to the next higher level of supervision.
- Evaluate the resources required for the treatment of patients and report the needs to next level of command.
- Identify and establish suitable "immediate care" and "delayed care" treatment areas and an ambulatory patient assembly area.
- Assign and coordinate the resources necessary to provide suitable treatment for all patients, and provide site safety for all patients and rescuers.
- Supervise assigned resources, treatment teams, medical supply personnel, litter bearers, hospital response teams, on-site physician help, etc.
- Ensure that all arriving patients have been or will be triaged.
- Provide for continuing evaluation and reassessment of patients' conditions.
- Determine the transportation priorities for patients.
- Give frequent and timely progress reports to Command.
- Coordinate activities with other operating units and groups as needed.
- Maintain incident documentation.
- Report to the next higher level of supervision when all patients have been moved from the treatment area(s) to the transportation area or other designated locations.
- Terminate treatment area activities and reallocate assigned resources as directed by next higher level of supervision.

Transportation Function

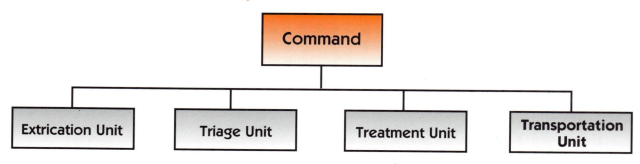

The Transportation Unit is responsible for determining and arranging all of the transportation needs for a multiple-patient incident. The Transportation Unit is also responsible for patient allocation to medical facilities in consultation with the Treatment Unit Leader and medical facilities.

The Transportation Unit Leader is appointed by the Incident Commander to establish a site to manage patient transportation from the scene to appropriate medical facilities. The Transportation Unit Leader must "size up" the transportation needs. All requests for transportation resources must be communicated to the next higher level of supervision. Command will then order the required resources. Once resources are on the scene and assigned to the Transportation Unit, they will report to the Transportation Unit Leader for further direction.

The Transportation Unit Leader must ensure that contact with appropriate medical facilities is accomplished as soon as possible to determine the facility's capabilities to receive patients. The initial notification should include an advisory of the incident situation and a request to determine the medical facility's treatment capability. The advisory should include type of incident, location of incident, total estimate of the number of patients, and some estimates of the number of patients by triage category. Additional information should be forwarded as more accurate information is obtained and time permits. Hospital specialty must be considered in treatment capability and patient allocation.

Medical control hospitals must be advised of the emergency medical incident situation as standing orders will be the primary method of treating advanced life support patients. Most trauma-related incidents will require very rapid treatment, using standard medical procedures, followed by prompt transport.

The Treatment Unit advises the Transportation Unit when each patient is ready for transport. The Transportation Unit allocates these patients to medical facilities based on patient injury and priority, hospital capacity and specialty, and by available transportation modes.

Transportation personnel pickup patients from the treatment area when they are ready for transport, and deliver them to the selected ambulances or other transportation conveyances. Patients should not be removed from the treatment area until they are ready for transport. Transportation and Treatment Unit personnel must maintain close coordination to determine the most appropriate allocation for each patient.

The Transportation Unit Leader must assume a visible position in the area. Management of this function may require additional resources to assist the Transportation Unit Leader based on the number of patients to be transported and the complexity of the incident. Additional personnel may be needed for medical communications, transport loading, ground medical transport coordination, record keeping, air medical transport coordination, and ambulance staging.

In complex incidents or geographically difficult areas, establishing a specific Staging Area for medical transportation may be necessary. It may also be necessary for ambulances or other vehicles to transport patients to an air operations landing zone.

The Transportation Unit Leader should be located close to the Treatment Unit Leader since frequent communications and coordination will be necessary between these two individuals. Effective transportation operations will require at least two (2) radio channels. Communication between the Transportation Unit and hospitals must be established on a separate radio channel that is used by the Medical Communications Manager. This will avoid interference with the tactical channel that is used by the Incident Commander. The Transportation Unit Leader must also maintain communications with Command on the tactical channel.

As patients are loaded into ambulances, triage tag stubs must be removed and delivered to the Medical Communications Manager. Stubs are used to advise hospitals of inbound patients and to maintain an accounting of all patient destinations.

Hospitals must be updated with patient information as time and information permits. As patients are transported from the scene, the hospitals should be advised of the estimated arrival time and of basic patient information.

All ambulances must be staged off site and brought in as needed. Ambulances should go to a single central staging area (preferably the same Staging Area for all resources responding to the incident) and brought to the scene one or two at a time for patient loading. In some situations, a separate ambulance staging area may be required. A Staging Area Manager will be required for each.

The Transportation Unit Leader's responsibilities can be summarized as follows:

- Determine the transportation requirements for all patients.
- Report resource and transportation requirements to the next higher level of supervision.
- Obtain the necessary transportation needs.
- Identify ambulance staging and helicopter landing zones if needed.
- Communicate with medical facilities to determine treatment capability.
- Coordinate patient transportation and allocation with the Treatment Unit.

- Supervise the movement of the patients from the treatment area to ambulance loading areas or helicopter landing zones.
- Notify the hospital and give them updates.
- Maintain accurate accounting of all patients and patient destinations.
- Coordinate with other tactical level management units.
- Maintain incident documentation.
- Alert all hospitals when the last patient is transported and the transportation function is terminated.

The organizational chart below illustrates the basic command organization that is established with the initial "first wave" response of resources. This organization may effectively manage approximately 12 to 20 patients.

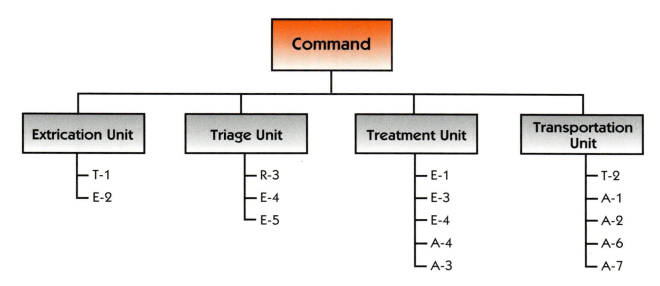

Expanded Organization — Reinforced Response for Emergency Medical Incidents

Staging Function

For major incidents, a reinforced response of additional alarms or mutual aid may be required. When this occurs, the command organization expands accordingly to manage the incident. One of the first additional command positions to be implemented is the Staging Area Manager. The scene can rapidly become very congested with unrequested apparatus responding directly to the impact area. To avoid this situation,

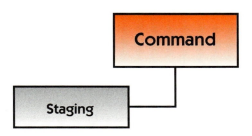

maximum control, coordination, communication, and direction of responding resources are imperative. As additional resources are requested, they must be directed to a Staging Area. Once in Staging, Command can direct companies or personnel to appropriate positions, often leaving apparatus in Staging or other out-of-the-way locations.

The Staging Area Manager's responsibilities can be summarized as follows:

- Determine an appropriate location for the Staging Area. Coordinate with the ambulance staging area if established.

- Coordinate staging activities with law enforcement representatives.

- Announce the Staging Area location to Command and Dispatch, and ensure that inbound companies are aware of routing to the Staging Area.

- Ensure that all apparatus are positioned properly in Staging to allow ease of exit. Drivers assigned for ambulance transport must be identified and readily available for dispatch to the transportation loading area.

- Assume a visible position. The Staging Area Manager should wear a vest that identifies him/her as such. All apparatus in Staging should turn off their emergency lights except for the Staging Area Manager's vehicle.

- Inventory all specialized equipment and report listing to Command. Establish a medical supply area if needed and requested.

- Give regular progress reports to Command (i.e. units remaining in staging, special equipment, etc.).

Note: Any responding agencies, organizations, groups, or individuals other than the first and reinforced response must report to Staging for assignments. This includes hospital response teams, physicians, and other allied health agencies or services.

Medical Group/Sector Function: Tactical Level Management Unit Expansion

For incidents involving a very large number of patients, or as the command organization continues to expand, a Medical Group/Sector Supervisor may be added to the organization as the initial step in establishing the medical function. This is done as a span-of-control mechanism to supervise the expanding responsibilities of the Triage, Treatment, and Transportation Units. It may also be established by the Incident Commander in the early stages of an incident that may not initially contain casualties but that has that potential to produce mass casualties before it is through.

The establishment of the Medical Group Supervisor will free up the next level of command established and allow for more control, coordination and communications with the established medical units, the transportation unit and with the Operations Section Chief or Command. In other situations, a Medical Branch (see chapter 4) may be preferred to provide this supervision and multiple Medical Groups are formed with a central patient transportation group. The Transportation Unit Leader would then be moved up to a Group Supervisor.

When the Medical Group Supervisor position is established, all supporting positions of the emergency medical function (Triage, Treatment, and Transportation Units) report to the Medical Group Supervisor. If the medical supply function was established under Treatment Unit or Staging, that function moves under the Group Supervisor and becomes a Unit Leader.

The Medical Group Supervisor's responsibilities may be summarized as follows:

- Ensure that the functions of triage, treatment, and transportation are carried out.
- Supervise and coordinate the Triage, Treatment, and Transportation Unit functions and personnel assigned.
- Determine/request resource needs.
- Communicate resource needs to Command.
- Recommend the expansion of the command organization as needed.
- Communicate direction and objectives to groups/units.
- Ensure that all units are completing objectives and responsibilities.
- Maintain incident documentation.

Additional Positions Within the Medical Group

Depending on the scope and severity of the incident, there are a number of other positions that may need to be implemented within the Medical Group. These positions include:

- Immediate/Delayed/Minor Treatment Managers
- Treatment Dispatcher Manager
- Medical Communications Manager/Coordinator
- Medical Supply Unit Manager/Unit Leader
- Transport Recorder/Ground Ambulance Coordinator

- Transport Loader(s)
- Morgue Manager

Immediate/Delayed/Minor Treatment Managers

For major incidents involving very large numbers of patients, and the treatment area fills with more and more patients, the Treatment Unit Leader should appoint managers to supervise the immediate, delayed, and minor treatment areas. This is done as a span-of-control mechanism.

The Immediate/Delayed/Minor Treatment Manager's responsibilities may be summarized as follows:

- Ensure that proper ALS/BLS equipment and resources are requested from Treatment Unit Leader.
- Supervise assigned medical teams in treatment area, and ensure that appropriate medical care is provided.
- Notify Treatment Unit Leader when patients are ready for transport.

Treatment Dispatch Manager

For major incidents involving large numbers of patients, the Treatment Unit Leader will need assistance in managing patient readiness for transport. The Treatment Dispatch Manager works for and reports to the Treatment Unit Leader.

The Treatment Dispatch Manager's responsibilities may be summarized as follows:

- Establish communications with the Treatment and Transportation Unit Leaders.
- Verify that patients are transported in an appropriate priority order.
- Coordinate patient loading.

Medical Communications Manager

When the emergency medical incident has expanded because of the number of patients and complexity of the incident, the Transportation Unit Leader should assign a Medical Communications Manager to manage the medical communications requirements. That person is assigned to the Transportation Unit Leader.

The Medical Communications Manager's responsibilities can be summarized as follows:

- Establish and maintain communications with medical facilities.
- Determine and maintain current status of medical facility availability and capability.
- Communicate medical facility availability to the Transportation Unit Leader.
- Advise the medical facility of inbound patients and their estimated time of arrival (ETA).
- Maintain appropriate incident documentation, via the tracking system, relating to the location of patients transported from the scene, transporting triage status, and the unit transporting the patient.

Transport Recorder/Ground Ambulance Manager

When the emergency medical incident has expanded because of the number of patients and the complexity of the incident, the Transportation Unit Leader should assign a Transport Recorder/Ground Ambulance Manager. This person reports to the Transportation Unit Leader. This person is assigned to the ambulance loading area to meet arriving ambulance crew members.

The Transport Recorder/Ground Ambulance Manager's responsibilities can be summarized as follows:

- Maintain appropriate incident documentation, via the tracking system, relating to the location of patients transported from the scene, transporting triage status, and the ambulance transporting the patient.
- Coordinate and direct patient destination with departing ground ambulances based on Medical Communications Manager information.
- Request the appointment of one or more transport loaders if necessary.

Transport Loader(s)

The Transport Loader(s) is/are assigned to the ambulance loading area to meet the arriving ambulance crew members and escort them to the patient they will be responsible for transporting to the hospital. This person may also be responsible for moving patients from the treatment area to the transportation area.

Medical Supply Unit Leader

Major incidents will rapidly consume standard complements of medical supplies carried on apparatus. Additional supplies must be obtained and delivered to the site. This position is initially established under the Treatment Unit as a manager function, then becomes a Unit Leader when a Medical Group Supervisor is appointed by Command.

The Medical Supply Unit Leader's responsibilities can be summarized as follows:

- Acquire medical supplies and equipment, and maintain them on site.
- Request additional supplies from next higher level of supervision.
- Distribute medical supplies to operating companies.

Morgue Manager

The management of fatalities normally falls under the duties of the Triage Unit Leader. When indicated by the complexities of the incident, an experienced person should be assigned the function of Morgue Manager. This is for the temporary establishment of a morgue area or for securing the remains until appropriate relief by the jurisdiction's medical examiner/coroner's office.

The Morgue Manager's responsibilities may be summarized as follows:

- Request resources, aides, and litter bearers as needed.
- Control access into morgue area.
- Establish and secure morgue area or maintain secure area in the impact area (isolate away from any treatment area).
- Request medical examiner response to incident scene (per local SOPs).
- Identify body locations and identities if available. Maintain records by numbering, photographing, and drawing of location found (grid). Secure personal effects and keep belongings with remains.
- Consider storage of remains; request resources to assist with this function.
- Coordinate functions with law enforcement, and assist medical examiner's office.
- Provide progress reports to next higher level of supervision established to manage this function.

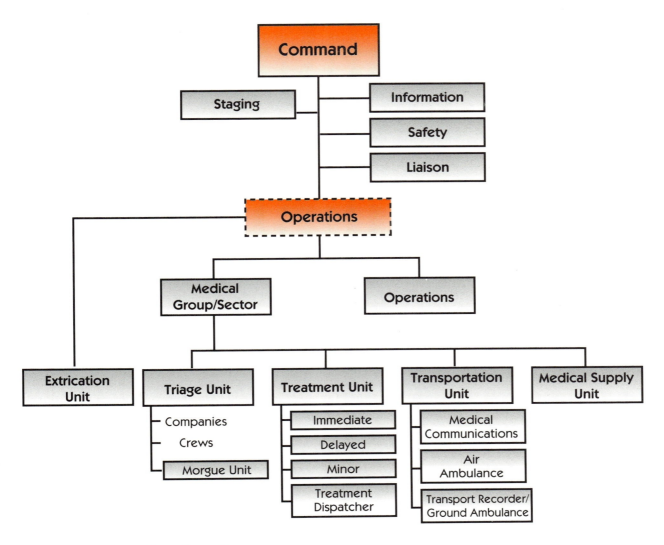

Air Operations/Landing Zone

Major incidents may require the use of air medical transport. A safe, designated landing location must be established. A person must be appointed to establish and manage the Air Operations/Landing Zone functions. Additional companies or units will be needed to staff and support the air operations functions.

Summary

It should be noted that as the Incident Management System expands to a major organization, so does the need for additional radio channels to support the operation, as well as more frequent face-to-face communication.

With this basic organization in place, the Incident Management System can easily manage any large number of patients and can expand further to disaster level operations. All the needed tactical level management units are in place. The only difference with larger numbers of patients is that each functioning element will be managing more patients and will be provided additional companies or crews to carry out their function. This will require greater supervision and tactical level management coordination of resources. Ultimately, this will lead the Incident Commander to establishing branch level operations into the command structure. Branch level operations are covered in more detail in Chapter 4 of this manual.

4

Command Structure – Branches

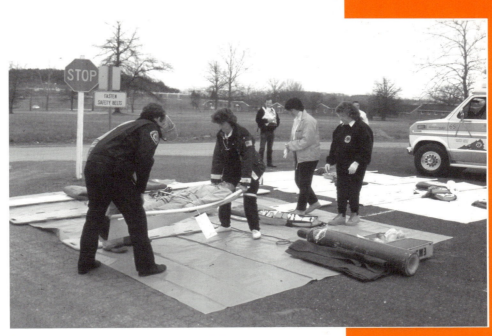

Photo courtesy of Virginia Office of EMS

4

Command Structure — Branches

Expanding the Organization — Branches

As an event escalates into a major incident, additional organizational support will be required. The Incident Commander can become quickly overwhelmed and overloaded with information management, assigning companies, filling out and updating the tactical work sheets, planning, forecasting, requesting additional resources, talking on the radio, and fulfilling all the other functions of Command. The immediate need of the Incident Commander is support. As additional ranking officers arrive on the scene, the command organization may be expanded through the involvement of officers and staff personnel filling Command and General Staff positions.

Section level positions can be implemented at any time, based on the needs of the incident. One of the first positions typically implemented is the Operations Section Chief. This is covered in more detail in Chapter 5 of this manual.

Branches

As previously discussed in this document, divisions/groups or sectors identify tactical level management assignments in the command structure. The organization can be further subdivided into Branches when:

- The span of control begins to be excessive.
- The incident becomes more complex (i.e., multi-jurisdictional, worsening conditions)
- The incident has two or more distinctly different operations (i.e., fire, medical, law enforcement).

Branches may be established at an incident to serve several purposes. However, they are not always essential to the organization of the Operations Section. When the numbers of divisions/groups or sectors exceed the recommended span of control, the Incident Commander or Operations Section Chief should designate a multi-branch structure, and allocate the tactical level management units within those branches.

In the following example, the Incident Commander has one group and four divisions reporting with two additional divisions and one group being added. This will exceed established span-of-control limits. At this point, a branch organization should be formed.

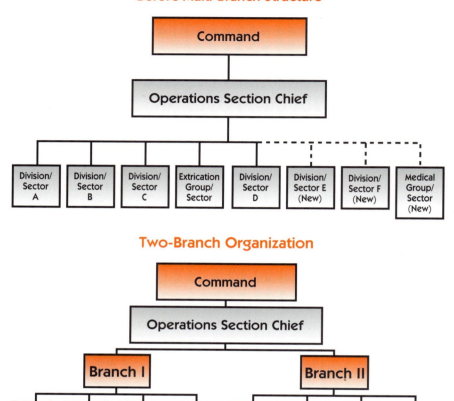

Branches should operate in their area of responsibility on separate radio channels, and communicate to Command or Operations on a different channel if possible. When designating functional branches, the radio designation of branches should reflect the objective of the branch, (i.e., Fire Branch, Medical Branch). Tactical branches may be designated numerically (i.e., Branch I, Branch II, Branch III).

When the Incident Commander implements Branch Directors, the tactical level management unit supervisors should be notified of their new supervisor. This information should include:

- What branch the division/group or sector is now assigned to.
- The radio channel those branch elements are operating on.

Radio communications should then be directed from the tactical level management unit supervisor to the Branch Director, instead of Command or Operations. Supervisors will relay information on the branch formation to the companies operating in their assigned area.

Three-Branch Organization

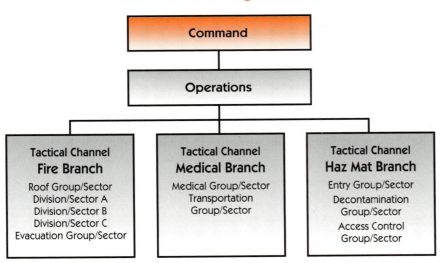

Depending on the situation, Branch Directors may be located at the command post or at operational locations. When located at the command post, Branch Directors can communicate on a face-to-face basis with the Operations Section Chief and/or Incident Commander.

When an incident encompasses a large geographic area, it may be more effective to have branches in tactical locations. When branches are sent to tactical positions, they should immediately implement command and control procedures within their branch. In these situations Operations must assign someone to monitor a branch radio command channel.

Branches are not limited to the Operations Section. Any of the section chiefs may recommend the implementation of branches within their sections with approval of the Incident Commander. This process is explained in further detail in Chapter 5 of this manual.

In the following example of an organization for a commercial airliner crash with multiple patients, fuel spillage, and a major fire, the Incident Commander has established the following tactical level management units with the "first wave" of resources:

Aircraft Crash Prior to Branch Implementation

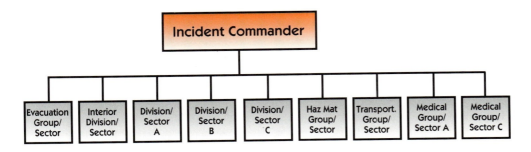

As the reinforced "second wave" of resources arrives, the Incident Commander recognizes a major, escalating incident, and splits the organization into manageable branches as illustrated below.

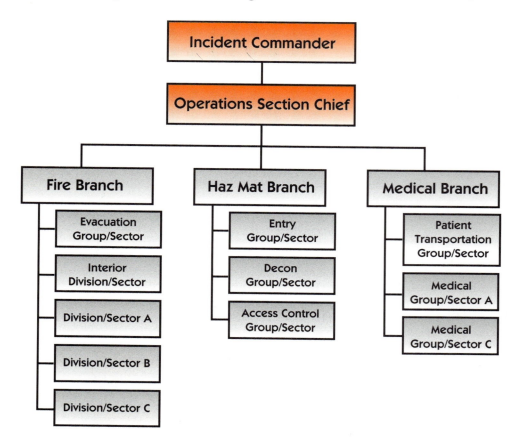

Functional Branch Structure

When the nature of the incident calls for a functional branch structure, such as a major aircraft crash within a jurisdiction involving police, fire, and medical departments, each has a functional branch operating under the direction of an Operations Section Chief. In this example, the Operations Section Chief is from the fire department, with Branch Directors from the fire, police, and medical services departments. Other alignments could be made depending upon the jurisdictional plan and type of emergency. Note that Command in this situation could be either Single or Unified Command depending upon the jurisdiction. Unified Command is covered in more detail in Chapter 6 of this manual.

When the incident is multi-jurisdictional, resources are best managed under the agencies that have normal control over them. Branches should be utilized at incidents where the span of control with tactical level management units are maximized — incidents involving two or more distinctly different major management compo-

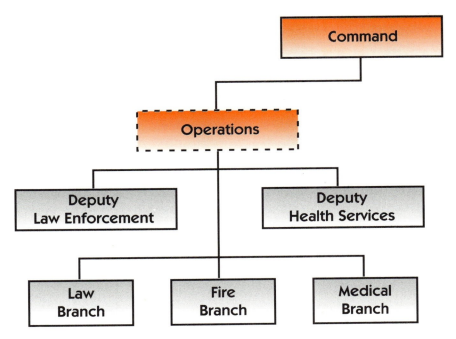

nents (i.e., a large fire with a major evacuation, a large fire with a large number of patients). The Incident Commander may elect to assign branches to forward positions to manage and coordinate activities.

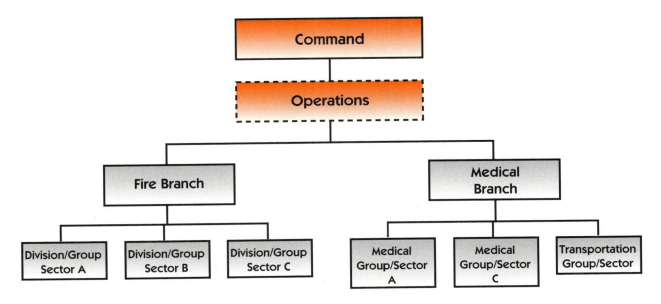

When the incident requires the use of aircraft, such as for the transportation of victims from an emergency medical incident, high-rise roof top rescue, swift water rescue, or a wildland fire, the Incident Commander or Operations Section Chief should establish the Air Operations organization. Its size, organization, and use will depend primarily upon the nature of the incident and the availability of aircraft.

Branches with Operations Section Chief Supervision

The Operations Section is most often implemented (staffed) as a span-of-control mechanism. When the number of branches or tactical level management units exceeds the capability of the Incident Commander to effectively manage, the Incident Commander may staff the Operations Section. This will reduce his/her span of control and thus transfer direct management of all tactical activities to the Operations Section Chief. The Incident Commander is then able to focus his/her attention on management of the entire incident rather than concentrating on tactical activities. Section level positions will be discussed in detail in Chapter 5.

5
Command Structure - Expanding the Organization

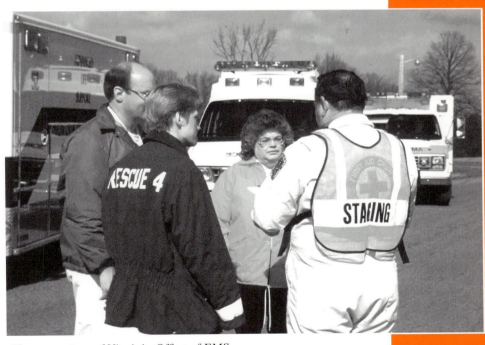
Photo courtesy of Virginia Office of EMS

5
Command Structure — Expanding the Organization

Expanding the Organization — Sections

As previously noted, when a small event escalates into a major incident, additional organizational support will be required. The Incident Commander can become quickly overwhelmed and overloaded with a variety of responsibilities related to the functions of Command.

Section and unit level positions within the Incident Management System will be activated only when the corresponding functions are required by the incident. Until such time as a section is activated, all functions associated with that section will be the responsibility of the Incident Commander or the appropriate Section Chief. It is recommended that two or more units not be combined into a single unit. However, an individual may be assigned responsibility for managing more than one unit. This method of organization allows for easy expansion and demobilization of the system.

The command structure defines the lines of authority, but it is not intended that the transfer of information within the Incident Management System be restricted to the chain of command. An individual will receive orders from a superior but may give information to any position in a different part of the organization within the guidelines specified in the operational procedures for each position.

The majority of positions within the Incident Management System will not be activated until the initial response is determined to be insufficient to handle the situation. When this occurs, additional resources are requested through normal dispatching procedures to fill the positions determined to be required for the type of incident in progress. If it is later determined that a specific position is not needed, the request can be canceled. Some agencies have elected to use a modular form of dispatching, such as dispatching entire units together.

The transition from the initial response to a major incident organization will be evolutionary, and positions will be filled as the corresponding tasks are required.

During the initial phases of the incident, the Incident Commander normally carries out these four section functions:

- Operations
- Planning
- Logistics
- Finance/Administration

These comprise the General Staff within a fully expanded incident organizational structure.

Operations Section

One of the first sections typically implemented is the Operations Section. The Operations Section is most often implemented (staffed) as a span-of-control mechanism. When the number of tactical level management units or branches exceed the capability of the Incident Commander to effectively manage, the Incident Commander may staff the Operations Section to reduce span of control and thus transfer direct management of all tactical activities to the Operations Section Chief. The Incident Commander is then able to focus attention on management of the entire incident rather than concentrating on tactical activities.

Operations Section Chief

The Operations Section Chief is responsible for the direct management of all incident tactical activities, the tactical priorities, and the safety and welfare of the personnel working in the Operations Section. The Operations Section Chief should have direct involve-

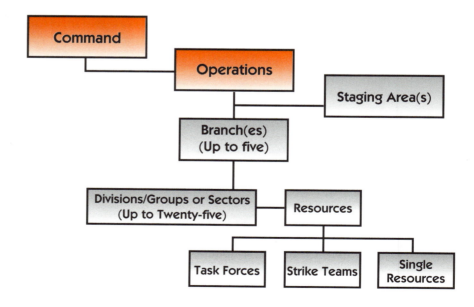

ment in the preparation of the action plan for the period of responsibility. The Operations Section Chief uses the appropriate radio channel to communicate strategic and specific objectives to the branches and/or tactical level management units.

The Operations Section Chief's responsibilities can be summarized as follows:

- Manage incident tactical activities.
- Coordinate activities with the Incident Commander.
- Implement the incident action plan.
- Assign resources to tactical level areas based on tactical objectives and priorities.
- Build an effective organizational structure through the use of branches and/or tactical level management units.
- Provide tactical objectives for tactical level management units.
- Control Staging and Air Operations.
- Provide for life safety.
- Determine needs and request additional resources.
- Consult with and inform other sections and the incident command staff as needed.

The Incident Commander's Role and Responsibilities After the Activation of an Operations Section Chief

Once the Operations Section is in place and functioning, the Incident Commander's focus should be on the strategic issues, overall strategic planning, and other components of the incident. This focus is to look at the "big picture" and the impact of the incident from a broad perspective. The Incident Commander should provide direction, advice, and guidance to the Command and General Staff in directing the tactical aspects of the incident.

The Incident Commander's role and responsibilities after the Operations Section is implemented are:

- Review and evaluate the incident action plan, and initiate any needed changes.
- Provide on-going review of the overall incident (THE BIG PICTURE).
- Select priorities.
- Provide direction to the Command and General Staff.
- Review the organizational structure; initiate change or expansion to meet incident needs.

- Staff Command and General Staff functions as necessary.
- Establish liaison with other internal agencies and officials, outside agencies, property owners, and/or tenants.

Staging Areas

The incident scene can quickly become congested with emergency equipment unless this equipment is managed effectively. Staging Areas are locations designated within the incident area to temporarily locate resources available for assignment. For major or complex operations, the Incident Commander should establish a central Staging Area early and place an officer in charge of staging. The radio designation "Staging" should be utilized.

In the expanded organizational structure, Staging reports to the Operations Section Chief. The Operations Section Chief may establish, move, or discontinue the use of Staging Areas. All resources within the designated Staging Areas are under the direct control of the Operations Section Chief and should be immediately available. Staging will request any logistical support they may require (food, fuel, sanitation, etc.) from the Logistics Section.

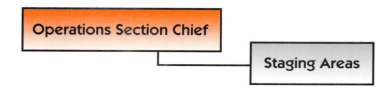

Planning Section

The Planning Section is responsible for gathering, assimilating, analyzing, and processing information needed for effective decision making. Information management is a full-time task at large and complex incidents. The Planning Section serves as the Incident Commander's "clearinghouse" for information. This allows the Incident Commander's staff to provide information instead of having to deal with dozens of information sources. Critical information should be immediately forwarded to Command (or whoever needs it). Information should also be used to make long-range plans. The Planning Section Chief's goal is to plan ahead of current events and to identify the need for resources before they are needed.

The Planning Section Chief's responsibilities can be summarized as follows:

- Evaluate current strategy, and plan with the Incident Commander.
- Maintain resource status and personnel accountability.

- Refine and recommend any needed changes to the plan with Operations input.
- Evaluate incident organization and span of control.
- Forecast possible outcome(s).
- Evaluate future resource requirements.
- Utilize technical assistance as needed.
- Evaluate tactical priorities, specific critical factors, and safety.
- Gather, update, improve, and manage situation status with a standard systematic approach.
- Coordinate with any needed outside agencies for planning needs.
- Plan for incident demobilization.
- Maintain incident records.

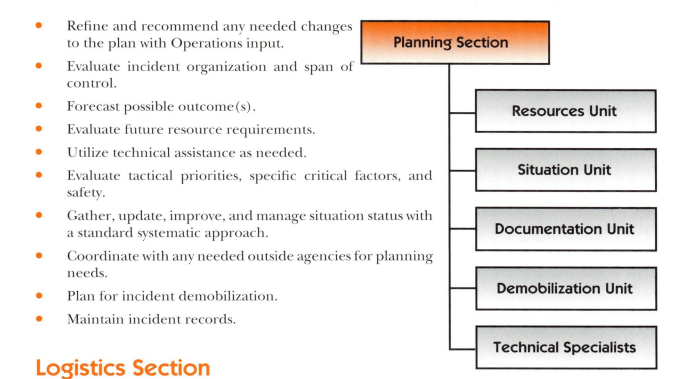

Logistics Section

The Logistics Section is the support mechanism for the organization. Logistics provides services and support systems to all the organizational components involved in the incident including facilities, transportation, supplies, equipment maintenance, fueling, feeding, communications, and medical services, including responder rehabilitation.

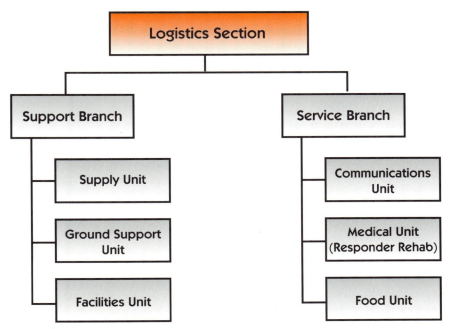

The responsibilities of the Logistics Section can be summarized as follows:

- Provide for requested medical aid for incident personnel, and manage responder rehabilitation.
- Coordinate immediate critical incident stress debriefing function.
- Provide and manage any needed supplies or equipment.
- Forecast and obtain future resource needs (coordinate with the Planning Section).
- Provide for the communications plan and any needed communications equipment.
- Provide fuel and needed repairs for equipment.
- Obtain specialized equipment or expertise per Command.
- Provide food and associated supplies.
- Secure any needed fixed or portable facilities.
- Provide any other logistical needs as requested by Command.
- Supervise assigned personnel.

Finance/Administration Section

The Finance/Administration Section is established on incidents when the agency(ies) involved have a specific need for financial services. Not all agencies will require the establishment of a separate Finance/Administration Section. In some cases where only one specific function is required, such as cost analysis, that position could be established as a Technical Specialist in the Planning Section.

The responsibilities of the Finance/Administration Section can be summarized as follows:

- Procure services and/or supplies from sources within and outside the fire department or city as requested by Command (coordinates with Logistics).
- Document all financial costs of the incident.
- Document cost recovery information for services and/or supplies.
- Analyze and manage legal risk for incidents (i.e., hazardous materials cleanup).
- Document for compensation and claims for injury.

The Finance/Administration Section is responsible for obtaining any and all needed incident documentation for potential cost recovery efforts.

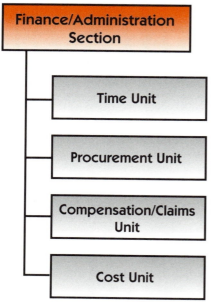

Incident Command Staff

Command staff positions are established to assume responsibility for key activities that are not a part of the line organization. Three specific staff positions are identified:

- Information Officer
- Safety Officer
- Liaison Officer

Additional positions might be required, depending upon the nature and location of the incident or by requirements established by Incident Command.

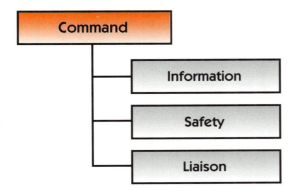

Information Officer

The Information Officer's function is to develop accurate and complete information regarding incident cause, size, current situation, resources committed, and other matters of general interest. The Information Officer will normally be the point of contact for the media and other governmental agencies which desire information directly from the incident. In either a Single or Unified Command structure, only one Information Officer would be designated. Assistants may be assigned from other agencies or departments involved.

Safety Officer

The Safety Officer's function at the incident is to assess hazardous and unsafe situations, and develop measures for assuring personnel safety. The Safety Officer has emergency authority to stop and/or prevent unsafe acts. In a Unified Command structure, a single Safety Officer would be designated. Assistants may be required and may be assigned from other agencies or departments making up the Unified Command. The Safety Officer may be involved in determining the need for responder rehabilitation.

Liaison Officer

The Liaison Officer's function is to be a point of contact for representatives from other agencies. In a Single Command structure, the representatives from assisting agencies would coordinate through the Liaison Officer. Under a Unified Command structure, representatives from agencies not involved in the Unified Command would coordinate through the Liaison Officer. Agency representatives assigned to an incident should have authority to speak on all matters for their agency.

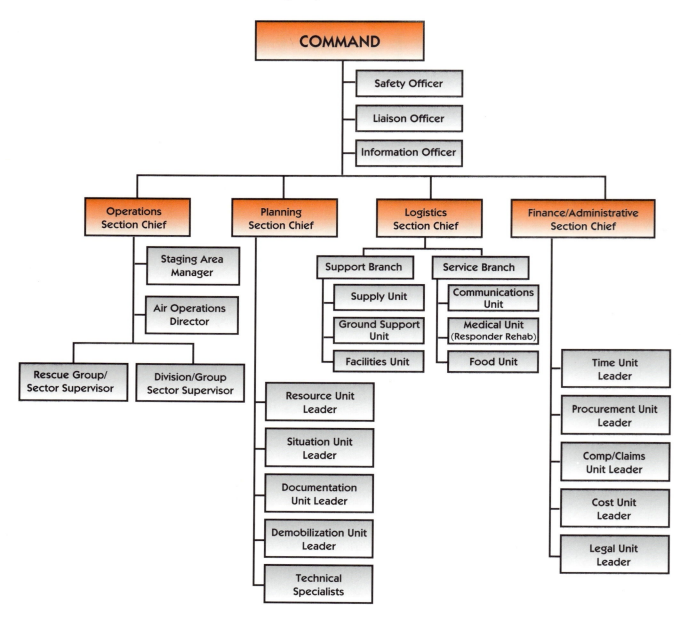

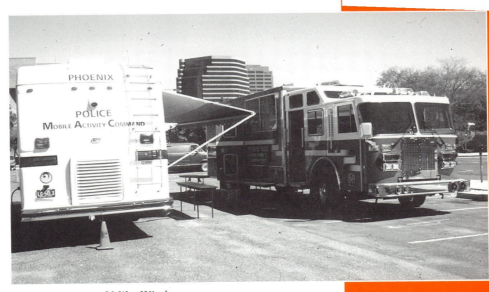

Photo courtesy of Mike Wieder

Unified Comm

6
Unified Command

Command is responsible for overall management of the incident. Command also includes certain staff functions. The Command function within the IMS may be conducted in two general ways:

- Single Command
- Unified Command

Single Command — Incident Commander

A single Incident Commander will be designated by the jurisdictional agency to have overall management responsibility for an incident that does not overlap jurisdictional boundaries.

The Incident Commander will prepare incident objectives that will serve as the foundation for subsequent action planning. The Incident Commander will approve the final action plan and approve all requests for the ordering and releasing of primary resources. The Incident Commander may have a deputy. The deputy should have the same qualifications as the Incident Commander. The deputy may work directly with the Incident Commander, be a relief Incident Commander, or perform certain specific assigned tasks.

At an incident within a single jurisdiction where the nature of the incident is primarily the responsibility of one agency; for example, fire, the deputy may be from the same agency. In a multi-jurisdictional incident, or one which threatens to be multi-jurisdictional, the deputy role may be filled by an individual designated by the adjacent agency. More than one deputy could be involved. Another way of organizing to meet multi-jurisdictional situations is described under Unified Command.

Single Incident Command Structure

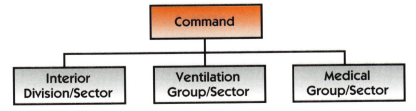

Unified Command

A Unified Command structure is called for under the following conditions:

- The incident is single jurisdiction multi-agency in nature due to the different kinds of resources required; e.g., a passenger airliner crash within a national forest. Fire, medical, and law enforcement all have immediate but diverse objectives. An example of this kind of Unified Command structure is depicted below.

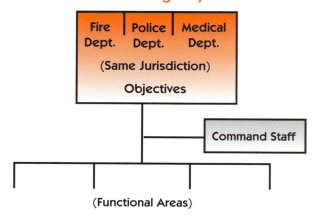

- The incident is multi-jurisdictional in nature; e.g., a major flood. An example of this Unified Command structure is shown below.

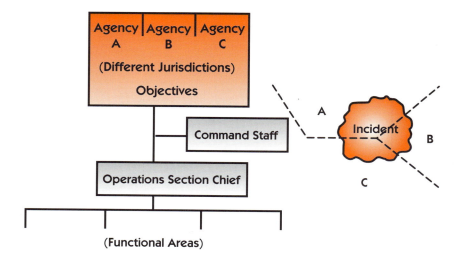

Single/Unified Command Differences

The primary differences between the Single and Unified Command structures are:

- In a Single Command structure, a single Incident Commander is solely responsible, within the confines of his/her authority, to establish objectives and overall management strategy associated with the incident. The Incident Commander is directly responsible for follow-through to ensure that all functional area actions are directed toward accomplishment of the strategy. The implementation of the planning required to effect operational control will be the responsibility of a single individual (Operations Section Chief) who will report directly to the Incident Commander.

- In a Unified Command structure, the individuals designated by either their jurisdictions or by departments within a single jurisdiction must jointly determine objectives, strategy, and priorities. As in a Single Command structure, the Operations Section Chief will have responsibility for implementation of the plan. The determination of which agency or department the Operations Section Chief represents must be made by mutual agreement of the Unified Command. It may be done on the basis of greatest jurisdictional involvement, number of resources involved, existing statutory authority, or mutual knowledge of the individual's qualifications.

Unified Command — Integrating Non-Fire Service EMS Agencies

Many communities have a non-fire service EMS agency that provides patient transportation and/or advanced life support services to the community. The term "third service" is used to describe an EMS agency that is independent of police or fire department management. A third service EMS agency may be another agency of the local or state government, or it may be a private, contract provider. Because the third service EMS agency is not normally managed by the fire department, when responding to an emergency medical incident it must be integrated into a Unified Command structure. There are several options and organizational designs with which to accomplish the integration.

Option 1. Absorbing EMS agency personnel

Using this option, the fire department assumes responsibility for all organizational positions. Personnel from the EMS agency are assigned to various tactical level management units as needed. The EMS personnel work for and are supervised by any qualified person appointed by Command to their assigned tactical management level unit.

Option 2. Use of a Medical Group or Branch

In this option, the first supervisor of the EMS agency on the scene is assigned the Medical Group responsibility. This supervisor implements and directs the Treatment and Transportation functions. Personnel from the EMS agency are assigned primarily to these areas. The basic organization and the positions described previously continue to be implemented as needed. However, it is absolutely essential that all command organizational positions have direct communication with the Incident Commander on the assigned tactical channel. Another approach may utilize a fire department officer in this position to supervise the assigned EMS resources.

Option 3. Integrating into existing positions

In this option, supervisors from the EMS agency may be assigned to assume any of the tactical level management unit positions they are qualified to manage. For example, the fire department may have officers assigned to extrication, staging, and landing zone responsibilities. The EMS agency may have officers managing triage, treatment, and transportation.

The options listed above are for operational as well as for planning purposes and should be addressed as needed by each jurisdiction adopting the Incident Management System.

Note: In order to be effective, all persons assuming organizational positions (i.e. group, sector) **must** have a portable radio that allows **direct** radio communications with Command or the Operations Section Chief.

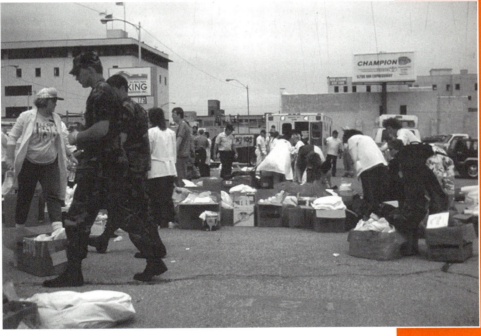
Photo courtesy of Mike Wieder

Appendices

A
Glossary of Terms

Advanced Life Support (ALS) — The level of emergency medical care that utilizes basic life support measures, invasive medical procedures, and drug therapy.

Agency Representative — Individual assigned to an incident from an assisting or cooperating agency who has been delegated full authority to make decisions on all matters affecting that agency's participation at the incident. Agency representatives report to the Incident Liaison Officer.

Allocated Resources — Resources dispatched to an incident that have not yet checked in with the Incident Commander.

ALS — *See* Advanced Life Support.

Ambulance — A ground vehicle providing patient transport capability, specified equipment capability, and personnel (basic life support ambulance or advanced life support ambulance, etc.).

Assigned Resources — Resources checked in and assigned work tasks on an incident.

Assisting Agency — An agency directly contributing suppression, rescue, support, or service resources to another agency.

Available Resources — Resources assigned to an incident and available for an assignment.

Base — That location at which the primary logistics functions are coordinated and administered. (Incident name or other designator will be added to the term "Base.") The incident command post may be co-located with the base. There is only one base per incident.

Basic Life Support (BLS) — The level of emergency medical care that involves maintenance of the patient's airway, breathing, and circulation. This level of care also includes basic bandaging and splinting of traumatic injuries.

Branch — That organizational level having functional/geographic responsibility for major segments of incident operations. The Branch level is organizationally between Section and Division/Sector/Group.

Brush Patrol — A light, mobile vehicle having limited pumping and water capacity for off-road operations.

Casualty Collection Point — A designated area for the control, processing, and triage of patients near an incident site or impact area.

APPENDIX A

Chief — IMS title for individuals responsible for command of the functional sections: Operations, Planning, Logistics, and Finance/Administration.

Clear Text — The use of plain English in radio communications transmissions. No ten codes or agency specific codes are used when using Clear Text.

Command Post (CP) — That location at which primary Command functions are executed, usually co-located with the Incident Base.

Command Staff — The Command Staff consists of the Information Officer, Safety Officer, and Liaison Officer, who report directly to the Incident Commander.

Command — The act of directing, ordering, and/or controlling resources by virtue of explicit legal, agency, or delegated authority.

Communications Unit — Functional unit within the Service Branch of the Logistics Section. This unit is responsible for the incident communications plan, the installation and repair of communications equipment, and operation of the incident communications center. Also may refer to a vehicle (trailer or mobile van) used to provide the major part of an incident communications center.

Company Unit Officer — The individual responsible for command of a company. This designation is not specific to any particular fire department rank (may be a firefighter, paramedic, lieutenant, captain, or chief officer, if responsible for command of a single company or ambulance).

Company — A ground vehicle providing specific equipment capability and personnel (engine company, truck company, rescue company, etc.).

Compensation/Claims Unit — Functional unit within the Finance/Administrative Section. Responsible for financial concerns resulting from injuries or fatalities at an incident.

Cooperating Agency — An agency supplying assistance other than direct suppression, rescue, support, or service functions to the incident control effort (Red Cross, law enforcement agency, telephone company, etc.).

Cost Unit — Functional unit within the Finance/Administration Section. Responsible for tracking costs, analyzing cost data, making cost estimates, and recommending cost-saving measures.

Crew — A specific number of personnel assembled for an assignment such as search, ventilation, or hoseline deployment and operations. The number of personnel in a crew should not exceed recommended span-of-control guides (3-7). A crew operates under the direct supervision of a Crew Leader.

Delayed Treatment — Secondary priority in patient treatment. Patients who fall into the delayed treatment classification require emergency medical care but not as urgently as those who are classified as "immediate treatment" patients.

Demobilization Unit — Functional unit within the Planning Section. Responsible for assuring orderly, safe, efficient demobilization of resources committed to the incident.

Director — IMS title for individuals responsible for command of a Branch.

Dispatch Center — A facility from which resources are directly assigned to an incident.

Division — That organizational level having responsibility for operations within a defined geographic area. The Division level is organizationally between single resources, task force, or the strike team and the Branch.

Documentation Unit — Functional unit within the Planning Section. Responsible for recording/protecting all documents relevant to incident.

Emergency Medical Technician (EMT) — Professional-level provider of basic or advanced life support emergency medical care. There are several classifications of EMTs depending on jurisdictional certification criteria, including:

    EMT-B — Basic Emergency Medical Technician

    EMT-CT — Emergency Medical Technician - Cardiac Technician

    EMT-D — Emergency Medical Technician - Defibrillator

    EMT-I — Emergency Medical Technician - Intermediate

    EMT-P — Emergency Medical Technician - Paramedic

Engine Company — A ground vehicle providing specified levels of pumping, water, hose capacity, and personnel.

Extrication Unit/Leader — An organizational position or function responsible for supervising the extrication of victims from entrapment and delivering them to a designated medical treatment area.

Facilities Unit — Functional unit within the Support Branch of the Logistics Section. Provides fixed facilities for the incident. These facilities may include the incident base, feeding areas, sleeping areas, sanitary facilities, and a formal command post.

Finance/Administration Unit — Responsible for all costs and financial actions of the incident. Includes the Time Unit, Procurement Unit, Compensation/Claims Unit, and the Cost Unit.

Food Unit — Functional unit within the Service Branch of the Logistics Section. Responsible for providing meals for personnel involved with the incident.

General Staff — The group of incident management personnel comprised of the Operations Section Chief, Planning Section Chief, Logistics Section Chief, and Finance/Administration Chief.

Ground Support Unit — Functional unit within the Support Branch of the Logistics Section. Responsible for fueling/maintaining/repairing vehicles and the transportation of personnel and supplies.

Group — That organizational level having responsibility for a specified functional assignment at an incident (ventilation, salvage, water supply, etc.).

Immediate Treatment — A patient who requires immediate assessment and medical intervention for survival.

Impact Area — The immediate area of an incident scene where the patients received their injuries and they were initially found.

Incident Action Plan — The strategic goals, tactical objectives, and support requirements for the incident. All incidents require an action plan. For simple incidents, the action plan is not usually in written form. Large or complex incidents will require that the action plan be documented in writing.

Incident Command System (ICS) — An Incident Management System with a common organizational structure with responsibility for the management of assigned resources to effectively accomplish stated objectives pertaining to an incident.

Incident Commander (IC) — The individual responsible for the management of all incident operations.

Information Officer — Responsible for interface with the media or other appropriate agencies requiring information direct from the incident scene. Member of the Command Staff.

Initial Attack — Resources initially committed to an incident.

Ladder Company — *See* Truck Company.

Leader — The individual responsible for command of a task force, strike team, or functional unit.

Liaison Officer — The point of contact for assisting or coordinating agencies. Member of the Command Staff.

Lobby Control — A control point for firefighting resources located in the lobby of a high-rise structure.

Logistics Section — Responsible for providing facilities, services, and materials for the incident. Includes the Communication Unit, Medical Unit, and Food Unit, within the Service Branch; and the Supply Unit, Facilities Unit, and Ground Support Unit, within the Support Branch.

Mass Casualty Incident — *See* Multi-Casualty Incident.

Medical Branch/Group/Sector — Organizational structure designed to provide the Incident Commander with a basic expandable system for handling the functions of triage, treatment, and transportation of patients in an emergency medical incident involving multiple casualties.

Medical Unit — Functional unit within the Service Branch of the Logistics Section. Responsible for providing emergency medical treatment of emergency personnel. This unit does not provide treatment for civilians.

Minor Treatment — Patients whose injuries are not severe and require only basic first aid intervention.

Morgue — An area on or near the incident site that is designated for the temporary placement of deceased victims. The Morgue is the responsibility of the Medical Examiner's/Coroner's Office once their representative is on the scene.

Multi-Casualty Incident — An emergency incident involving the injury or death of a number of patients beyond what the jurisdiction is routinely capable of handling. Also called Mass Casualty Incident.

Officer — The Command Staff positions of Safety, Liaison, and Information.

Operational Period — The period of time scheduled for execution of a given set of operation actions as specified in the incident action plan.

Operations Section — Responsible for all tactical operations at the incident. Includes up to 5 Branches, 25 Divisions/Groups/Sectors, and 125 single resources, task forces, or strike teams.

Out-of-Service Resources — Resources assigned to an incident but unable to respond for mechanical, rest, or personnel reasons.

Planning Meeting — A meeting held as needed throughout the duration of an incident to select specific strategies and tactics for incident control operations and for service and support planning.

Planning Section — Responsible for the collection, evaluation, dissemination, and use of information about the development of the incident and the status of resources. Includes the Situation Status, Resource Status, Documentation, and Demobilization Units as well as Technical Specialists.

Procurement Unit — A functional unit within the Finance/Administration Section. Responsible for financial matters involving vendors.

Rapid Intervention Crew (RIC) — A team or company designated to stand by in a state of readiness to effect rescues of firefighters who are in trouble.

Reporting Locations — Any one of six facilities/locations where incident-assigned resources may check in. The locations are: Incident Command Post — Resources Unit (RESTAT), Base, Camp, Staging Area, Helibase, or the Division Supervisor's location for direct line assignments. (Check in at one location only.)

Rescue Company — A ground vehicle providing specified rescue equipment, capability, and personnel.

Resource Status Unit (RESTAT) — Functional unit within the Planning Section. Responsible for recording the status of and accounting for resources committed to incident. Also responsible for the evaluation of resources currently committed to incident, the impact that additional responding resources will have on the incident, and anticipated resource needs.

Resources — All personnel and major items of equipment available, or potentially available, for assignment to incident tasks on which status is maintained.

Responder Rehabilitation (Rehab) — The function and/or location where medical evaluation and treatment, food and fluid replenishment, and relief from extreme climatic conditions are provided for emergency responders, according to the circumstances of the incident.

Safety Officer — Responsible for monitoring and assessing safety hazards and unsafe situations and developing measures for ensuring personnel safety. Member of the Command Staff.

Section — That organizational level having functional responsibility for primary segments of incident operations such as Operations, Planning, Logistics, and Finance/Administration. This Section level is organizationally between Branch and Incident Commander.

Section Chief — Title that refers to a member of the General Staff (Planning Section Chief, Operations Section Chief, Finance/Administration Section Chief, Logistics Section Chief).

Sector — A tactical level management unit having responsibility for either a geographic or functional assignment. Sector may take the place of either the Division or Group or both.

Service Branch — A branch within the Logistics Section. Responsible for service activities at incident. Components include the Communications Unit, Medical Unit, and Food Unit.

APPENDIX A

Single Resource — An individual company or crew.

Situation State Unit (SITSTAT) — Functional unit within the Planning Section. Responsible for analysis of situation as it progresses. Reports to Planning Section Chief.

Staging Area — That location where incident personnel and equipment are assigned on an immediately available status.

Stairwell Support — Personnel assigned to be responsible for the transportation of portable equipment from ground level to the staging floor of a high-rise structure.

Standing Orders — Policies and procedures approved by the local jurisdiction medical director for use by emergency medical personnel in situations where direct voice communications with the medical control hospital cannot be established or maintained.

START/S.T.A.R.T. — Acronym for Simple Triage and Rapid Treatment. This is a model initial triage system that has been adopted for use in many jurisdictions.

Strategic Goals — The overall plan that will be used to control the incident. Strategic goals are broad in nature and are achieved by the completion of tactical objectives.

Strike Team — Five of the same kind and type of resources with common communications and a leader.

Supervisor — Individuals responsible for command of a Division/Group/Sector.

Supply Unit — Functional unit within the Support Branch of the Logistics Section. Responsible for ordering equipment/supplies required for incident operations.

Support Branch — A branch within the Logistics Section. Responsible for providing the personnel, equipment, and supplies to support incident operations. Components include the Supply Unit, Facilities Unit, and Ground Support Unit.

Tactical Level Management Units — Term used to reference Divisions, Groups, or Sectors.

Tactical Objectives — The specific operations that must be accomplished to achieve strategic goals. Tactical objectives must be both specific and measurable.

Task Force — A group of any type or kind of resources with common communications and a leader; temporarily assembled for a specific mission (not to exceed five resources).

Technical Specialists — Personnel with special skills who are activated only when needed. Technical Specialists may be needed in the areas of fire behavior, water resources, environmental concerns, resource use, and training. Technical Specialists report initially to the Planning Section but may be assigned anywhere within the IMS organizational structure as needed.

Time Unit — Functional unit within the Finance/Administration Section. Responsible for record keeping of time for personnel working at incident.

Transportation Area — The area of the incident scene where patients are loaded into ambulances or to other vehicles for transfer to a medical facility.

Transportation Unit Leader — The person assigned to supervise the Transportation function under the Medical Group/Sector of the IMS organization.

Treatment Area — Specific area designated for the establishment of medical care to stabilize patients prior to transport to a medical facility. The areas include the Immediate, Delayed, and Minor Treatment areas.

Treatment Unit Leader — The person assigned to supervise the Treatment function under the Medical Group/Sector of the IMS organization.

Triage — The screening and classification of sick or injured persons to determine medical priority needs and to ensure effective and efficient use of medical personnel, equipment, and facilities.

Triage Unit Leader — The person assigned to supervise the Triage function under the Medical Group/Sector of the IMS organization.

Truck Company — A ground vehicle providing an aerial ladder or other aerial device and specified portable ladders and equipment along with required personnel.

Unit — That organizational element having functional responsibility for a specific incident's Planning, Logistics, or Finance/Administration activity.

B
Communications

Integrated communications at the incident are managed through the use of a common communications plan and an incident-based communications center established solely for the use of tactical and support resources assigned to the incident. All communications between organizational elements at an incident should be in plain English (also known as "clear text"). No codes should be used and all communications should be confined to essential messages only. The Communications Unit is responsible for all communications planning at the incident. This will include incident-established radio networks, on-site telephone, public address, and off-site telephone/microwave/radio systems.

Radio Networks

Radio networks for large incidents will normally be organized as follows:

Command Net

This net should link together Incident Command, key staff members, Section Chiefs, and tactical level management unit supervisors.

Tactical Nets

There may be several tactical nets. They may be established around agencies, departments, geographical areas, or even specific functions. The determination of how nets are set up should be a joint Planning/Operations Section function. The Communications Unit Leader will develop the plan.

Support Net

A support net will be established primarily to handle status changing for resources as well as for support requests and certain other nontactical or command functions.

Ground-to-Air Net

A ground-to-air net may be designated or regular tactical nets may be used to coordinate ground-to-air traffic.

Air-to-Air Net

Air-to-air nets will normally be predesignated and assigned for use at the incident.

C

Sample Triage Tags

METTAG Triage Tag

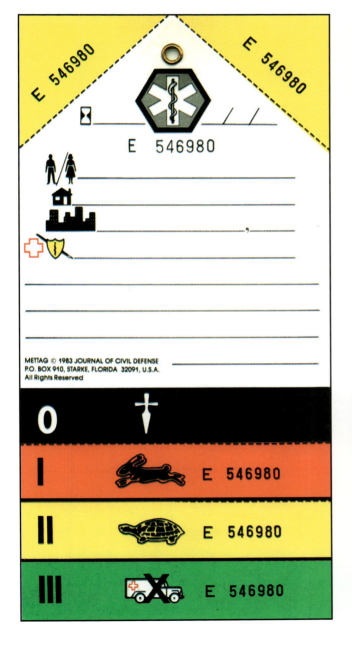
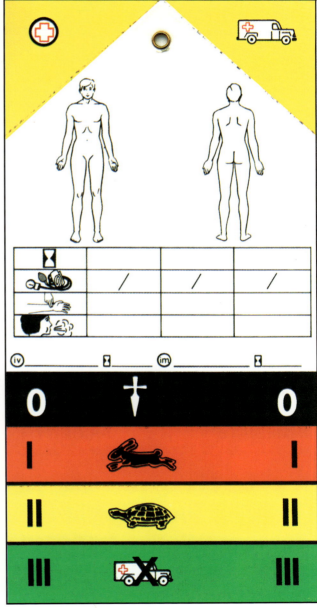

APPENDIX C

Phoenix Fire Department Triage Tags

Front:

92-23D Rev. 3/88

CITY OF PHOENIX, ARIZONA
FIRE DEPARTMENT

1 Nº 114163

IMMEDIATE PRIORITY

CO _____
NAME _____
AGE _____ INJURIES _____

TIME	PUPILS	BP	PULSE	RESP	SKIN

HOSPITAL _____
TREATMENT *(SEE BACK)*

- -

NAME _____
AMBULANCE _____
HOSPITAL _____

IMMEDIATE Nº 114163 **PRIORITY 1**

Back:

☐ UNCORRECTED RESPIRATORY PROBLEM
☐ CARDIAC ARREST
☐ SEVERE BLOOD LOSS
☐ UNCONSCIOUS
☐ SEVERE SHOCK
☐ OPEN CHEST or ABDOMINAL WOUNDS
☐ BURNS INVOLVE RESPIRATORY TRACT
☐ SEVERAL MAJOR FRACTURES

- -

TREATMENT _____

Phoenix Fire Department Triage Tags (continued)

92-24D Rev. 3/88

CITY OF PHOENIX, ARIZONA
FIRE DEPARTMENT

Nº 220773

2 DELAYED PRIORITY

CO_____

NAME_____

AGE_____ INJURIES_____

_____

TIME	PUPILS	BP	PULSE	RESP	SKIN

HOSPITAL_____

TREATMENT *(SEE BACK)*

- -

NAME_____

AMBULANCE_____

HOSPITAL_____

DELAYED   Nº 220773   **PRIORITY 2**

☐ SEVERE BURNS
☐ SPINAL COLUMN INJURIES
☐ MODERATE BLOOD LOSS
☐ CONSCIOUS WITH HEAD INJURIES
☐ MULTIPLE FRACTURES

- -

TREATMENT_____

_____

_____

_____

_____

Phoenix Fire Department Triage Tags (continued)

Tag 1 (front, left):

92-25D NEW 5/83 PHOENIX FIRE DEPARTMENT

№ 300841

3 AMBULATORY PATIENT

CO _____

NAME _____
AGE _____ INJURIES _____
_____
_____

TIME	PUPILS	BP	PULSE	RESP	SKIN

HOSPITAL _____
TREATMENT *(SEE BACK)* →

NAME _____
AMBULANCE _____
HOSPITAL _____

AMBULATORY PATIENT   № 300841   **PRIORITY 3**

Tag 2 (back, right):

☐ MINOR FRACTURES
☐ CONTUSIONS — ABRASIONS
☐ MINOR BURNS

TREATMENT _____
_____
_____
_____
_____

APPENDIX C

Phoenix Fire Department Triage Tags (continued)

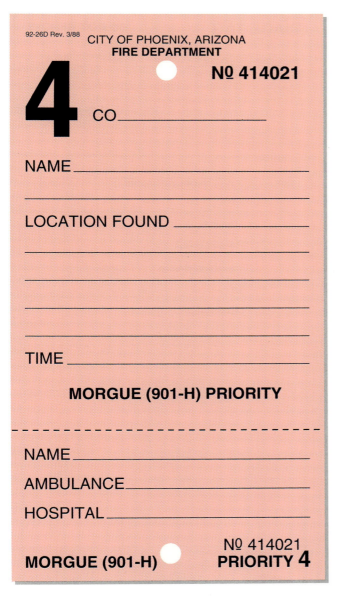
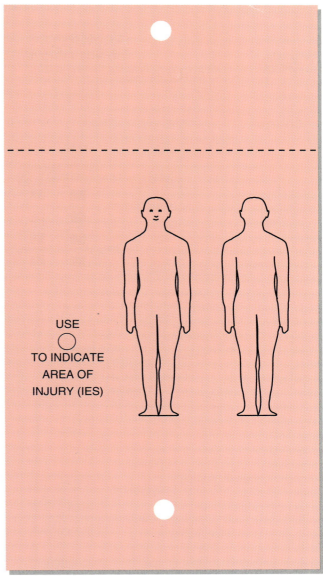

APPENDIX C

Commonwealth of Virginia Triage Tag

California Triage Tag

Triage Tag Part I

№ 115669

TRIAGE TAG PART I
№ 115669
CALIFORNIA FIRE CHIEF'S ASSOCIATION

FRONT — BACK

- C-SPINE
- CARDIAC
- BLUNT TRAUMA
- PENETRATING INJURY
- BURN
- FRACTURE
- LACERATION

OTHER _____

VITAL SIGNS:
ORIENTED ☐ DISORIENTED ☐ UNCONSCIOUS ☐

TIME	PULSE	B/P	RESPIRATION

DECEASED

IMMEDIATE № 115669

DELAYED № 115669

MINOR № 115669

Triage Tag Part II

TRIAGE TAG PART II

MEDICAL COMPLAINTS/HISTORY

ALLERGIES:
PATIENT R_x:

TIME	DRUG SOLUTION			DOSE
	D₅W	R/L	NS	

NOTES:

PERSONAL INFORMATION
NAME:
ADDRESS:
CITY: TEL. NO.:
MALE ☐   FEMALE ☐   AGE: WEIGHT:

DECEASED

IMMEDIATE

DELAYED

MINOR

For more information on the California tag, contact:

California Fire Chiefs Association
825 M Street
Rio Linda, CA 95673
(916) 445-9882

D

Sample Tactical Work Sheets for Emergency Medical Incidents

The sample tactical work sheets included on the following pages in this section are offered as examples from which a particular jurisdiction may be able to develop their own form.

D2

CITY OF PHOENIX, ARIZONA
FIRE DEPARTMENT
EMS MEDICAL WORKSHEET

☐ 2 + 1 MEDICAL
☐ FIRST ALARM MEDICAL

INCIDENT NO. _____

ADDRESS _____ TIME _____

INCIDENT TYPE _____

1️⃣ 2️⃣ 3️⃣ 4️⃣ 5️⃣ 6️⃣ 7️⃣ ☐

☐ INITIAL REPORT
☐ INITIATE COMMAND
☐ PERSONNEL PROTECTION
☐ TRIAGE
☐ EXTRICATION   ☐ ALL CLEAR
☐ TREATMENT
☐ TRANSPORTATION
☐ TRAFFIC/CROWD CONTROL
☐ HOSPITAL NOTIFICATION
☐ SCENE STABILIZED
☐ PROGRESS REPORTS
☐ _____

COMMAND

FIRE DEPT

EP	
EP	
EP	
E	
E	
L	
L	
R	
R	
BC	

RESCUE

1	
2	
3	
4	

HELICOPTER

1	
2	

EXTRICATION	TREATMENT	TRANSPORTATION	

PRIORITY 1	PRIORITY 2	PRIORITY 3	PRIORITY 4

PT# _____ PRIORITY _____
UNIT(S) TREATING _____
UNIT TRANSPORTING _____
HOSPITAL _____
INJURY _____
NAME _____
ADDRESS _____
SEX _____ AGE _____

PT# _____ PRIORITY _____
UNIT(S) TREATING _____
UNIT TRANSPORTING _____
HOSPITAL _____
INJURY _____
NAME _____
ADDRESS _____
SEX _____ AGE _____

PT# _____ PRIORITY _____
UNIT(S) TREATING _____
UNIT TRANSPORTING _____
HOSPITAL _____
INJURY _____
NAME _____
ADDRESS _____
SEX _____ AGE _____

PT# _____ PRIORITY _____
UNIT(S) TREATING _____
UNIT TRANSPORTING _____
HOSPITAL _____
INJURY _____
NAME _____
ADDRESS _____
SEX _____ AGE _____

PT# _____ PRIORITY _____
UNIT(S) TREATING _____
UNIT TRANSPORTING _____
HOSPITAL _____
INJURY _____
NAME _____
ADDRESS _____
SEX _____ AGE _____

PT# _____ PRIORITY _____
UNIT(S) TREATING _____
UNIT TRANSPORTING _____
HOSPITAL _____
INJURY _____
NAME _____
ADDRESS _____
SEX _____ AGE _____

APPENDIX D

CITY OF PHOENIX, ARIZONA
FIRE DEPARTMENT
TRANSPORTATION SECTOR

Treatment _____
LZ _____

AMBULATORY PATIENTS

VEHICLE	LOCATION	# OF PATIENTS

HELICOPTER I.D.
_____
_____
_____

Companies Assigned to Transportation
_____
_____
_____

- ❏ Med 9
- ❏ Sector Location
- ❏ Sector VEST
- ❏ LZ Location
- ❏ AMB STG Location
- ❏ TRIAGE Tag Stubs
- ❏ Command Progress Report
- ❏ Media Progress Report
- ❏ Last PT Trans.
- ❏ Resources
- ❏ Est. PT Total

PATIENT TRIAGE NUMBER	HOSP. _____ LEVEL _____	PRI 1	PRI 2	PRI 3	AMB I.D. #	PATIENT TRIAGE NUMBER	HOSP. _____ LEVEL _____	PRI 1	PRI 2	PRI 3	AMB I.D. #

PATIENT TRIAGE NUMBER	HOSP. _____ LEVEL _____	PRI 1	PRI 2	PRI 3	AMB I.D. #	PATIENT TRIAGE NUMBER	HOSP. _____ LEVEL _____	PRI 1	PRI 2	PRI 3	AMB I.D. #

D4

Sample 1

Tactical Worksheet

Address: _____ Incident No. _____ Time _____

Occupancy: _____

Wind Direction	**Personnel Accountability (PAR)**	Tactical	Benchmark	Functional
_____	All Clear	Overall Plan		Command Location
		Water Supply		Pumped Water
Elapsed Time	30 Min.	Search & Rescue		Gas
5 10 15 20 25 30 PAR		Initial Attack		Electrical
	Under Control	Exposures		Recon
		Rapid Intervention Team		Outside Agency
	Off-To-Def	Logistical Needs		Investigator
Level II Staging		Ventilation		P.P.V.
_____	Hazardous Event	Evacuation		P.D.
		All Clear		Primary-
	No "PAR" Upgrade Assign.	*Fire Control*		Secondary
		Salvage (Loss Stopped)		Salvage (Loss Stopped)
		Accountability		C.O. Meter

E
E
E
E
L
L
H
R
U
BC

E
E
E
E
L
L
H
R
U
BC

Branch — Command — Branch

APPENDIX D

COMMONWEALTH OF VIRGINIA
MASS CASUALTY INCIDENT MANAGEMENT TACTICAL WORKSHEET

COMMAND
- OFFICER
- RADIO CH
- LOCATION

OPERATIONS
- OFFICER
- RADIO CH
- LOCATION

EMS/MEDICAL CONTROL
- OFFICER
- LOCATION
- RADIO CH

POSITION	TIME	TIME	TIME	TIME	TIME
TRIAGE					
TREATMENT					
TRANSPORT					
MORGUE					

- INCIDENT #
- DATE
- TIME
- ADDRESS
- NATURE

TRIAGE
- OFFICER
- LOCATION
- RADIO CH
- TRIAGE TEAMS
- PORTER TEAMS

TREATMENT
- OFFICER
- LOCATION
- RADIO CH

IMMEDIATE TREATMENT	DELAYED TREATMENT	MINOR TREATMENT	MEDICAL SUPPLY
OFFICER	OFFICER	OFFICER	OFFICER
LOCATION	LOCATION	LOCATION	LOCATION
RADIO CH	RADIO CH	RADIO CH	RADIO CH
TREATMENT TEAMS	TREATMENT TEAMS	TREATMENT TEAMS	

TRANSPORTATION
- OFFICER
- LOCATION
- RADIO CH

TRANSPORT RECORDER
- OFFICER

TRANSPORT LOADER
- OFFICER

MEDICAL COMM	AMBULANC STAGING
OFFICER	OFFICER
RADIO CH	LOCATION / RADIO CH

HOSPITAL COMM	LOADING ZONE
PHYSICIAN	OFFICER
HOSPITAL	LOCATION / RADIO CH

MORGUE
- OFFICER
- LOCATION
- RADIO CH

EXTRICATION/RESCUE
- OFFICER
- LOCATION
- RADIO CH

TIME OR ✓ / TASKS

INITIAL
- SCENE SAFETY
- SCENE SURVEY
- 1st INITIAL BRIEFING
- EMS/MEDICAL CONTROL
- VANTAGE POINT
- ESTABLISH AMB STAGING
- PROVIDE STAGING INSTRUCTIONS
- MAKE ASSIGNMENTS

TRIAGE
- START TRIAGE TEAMS
- PORTER TEAMS

TREATMENT
- ESTABLISH TREATMENT AREAS
- SECONDARY TRIAGE
- SORT PATIENTS BY CATEGORY
- CONSIDER LIGHTING/ENVIRONMENT
- MEDICAL SUPPLIES
- ISOLATE EMOTIONALLY DISTURBED
- MOVE MINOR INJURIES TO OWN AREA

TRANSPORT
- ESTABLISH MEDICAL COMMUNICATIONS
- ALERT HOSPITALS
- STANDING ORDERS
- CONSIDER HELICOPTERS/LZ
- CONSIDER PATIENT/UNIT MOVEMENT

TERMINATION
- RELEASE UNITS ASAP
- NOTIFY HOSPITALS

RESOURCES

UNIT ID	STAFF	TIME IN	ASSIGNMENT #1	TIME OUT	READY	TIME IN	ASSIGNMENT #2	TIME OUT

CASUALTIES

INITIAL SURVEY — APPROXIMATE # PATIENTS — INJURIES: MAJOR _____ MINOR _____

TRIAGE REPORT TIME	UPDATES TIME	TIME	TIME	TIME	TIME	TIME	TOTAL TRANSPORTS
IMMEDIATE							
DELAYED							
MINOR							
DEAD							
TOTAL							

AREA HOSPITAL CAPABILITIES

FACILITY	CAPACITY			TRANSPORTED		
	IMMEDIATE	DELAYED	MINOR	IMMEDIATE	DELAYED	MINOR

APPENDIX D

D5

D6

OFFICER	COMMAND			COMMONWEALTH OF VIRGINIA		
RADIO CH	LOCATION			MASS CASUALTY INCIDENT MANAGEMENT		
OFFICER	OPERATIONS			TACTICAL WORKSHEET		
RADIO CH	LOCATION			IMMEDIATE/DELAYED/MINOR TREATMENT LOG		
OFFICER	EMS/MEDICAL CONTROL			INCIDENT #	SHEET ____ OF ____	
RADIO CH	LOCATION			DATE		
OFFICER	TREATMENT			TIME		
RADIO CH	LOCATION					
OFFICER	TRIAGE	OFFICER	TRANSPORTATION	ADDRESS		
RADIO CH	LOCATION	RADIO CH	LOCATION	NATURE		

#	PATIENT NAME/ TAG #	PRIMARY TRIAGE STATUS	TIME IN	SECONDARY TRIAGE STATUS	ASSESSMENT	TREATMENT	TIME OUT
1		IMMEDIATE DELAYED MINOR		IMMEDIATE DELAYED MINOR	PULSE _____ RESP _____ B/P _____ / _____ LOC _____ AVPU MEDICAL OR TRAUMA		
2		IMMEDIATE DELAYED MINOR		IMMEDIATE DELAYED MINOR	PULSE _____ RESP _____ B/P _____ / _____ LOC _____ AVPU MEDICAL OR TRAUMA		
3		IMMEDIATE DELAYED MINOR		IMMEDIATE DELAYED MINOR	PULSE _____ RESP _____ B/P _____ / _____ LOC _____ AVPU MEDICAL OR TRAUMA		
4		IMMEDIATE DELAYED MINOR		IMMEDIATE DELAYED MINOR	PULSE _____ RESP _____ B/P _____ / _____ LOC _____ AVPU MEDICAL OR TRAUMA		
5		IMMEDIATE DELAYED MINOR		IMMEDIATE DELAYED MINOR	PULSE _____ RESP _____ B/P _____ / _____ LOC _____ AVPU MEDICAL OR TRAUMA		
6		IMMEDIATE DELAYED MINOR		IMMEDIATE DELAYED MINOR	PULSE _____ RESP _____ B/P _____ / _____ LOC _____ AVPU MEDICAL OR TRAUMA		
7		IMMEDIATE DELAYED MINOR		IMMEDIATE DELAYED MINOR	PULSE _____ RESP _____ B/P _____ / _____ LOC _____ AVPU MEDICAL OR TRAUMA		
8		IMMEDIATE DELAYED MINOR		IMMEDIATE DELAYED MINOR	PULSE _____ RESP _____ B/P _____ / _____ LOC _____ AVPU MEDICAL OR TRAUMA		
9		IMMEDIATE DELAYED MINOR		IMMEDIATE DELAYED MINOR	PULSE _____ RESP _____ B/P _____ / _____ LOC _____ AVPU MEDICAL OR TRAUMA		
10		IMMEDIATE DELAYED MINOR		IMMEDIATE DELAYED MINOR	PULSE _____ RESP _____ B/P _____ / _____ LOC _____ AVPU MEDICAL OR TRAUMA		
11		IMMEDIATE DELAYED MINOR		IMMEDIATE DELAYED MINOR	PULSE _____ RESP _____ B/P _____ / _____ LOC _____ AVPU MEDICAL OR TRAUMA		
12		IMMEDIATE DELAYED MINOR		IMMEDIATE DELAYED MINOR	PULSE _____ RESP _____ B/P _____ / _____ LOC _____ AVPU MEDICAL OR TRAUMA		

APPENDIX D

COMMONWEALTH OF VIRGINIA
MASS CASUALTY INCIDENT MANAGEMENT TACTICAL WORKSHEET
TRANSPORTATION TACTICAL WORKSHEET

OFFICER	OPERATIONS
RADIO CH	LOCATION
OFFICER	EMS/MED CONTROL
RADIO CH	LOCATION
OFFICER	TRANSPORTATION
RADIO CH	LOCATION
OFFICER	MEDICAL COMMUNICATIONS
RADIO CH/PHONE #	LOCATION

DATE
TIME INCIDENT # SHEET____ OF ____
ADDRESS
NATURE

PATIENT NAME/ TAG #	TRIAGE STATUS IMMEDIATE DELAYED MINOR	NATURE OF COMPLAINT	HOSPITAL	UNIT TRANSPORTING	TIME OUT	OTHER

COMMONWEALTH OF VIRGINIA
MASS CASUALTY INCIDENT MANAGEMENT TACTICAL WORKSHEET
AMBULANCE STAGING WORKSHEET

OFFICER	COMMAND
RADIO CH	LOCATION
OFFICER	OPERATIONS
RADIO CH	LOCATION
OFFICER	EMS/MEDICAL CONTROL
RADIO CH	LOCATION
OFFICER	TRANSPORTATION
RADIO CH	LOCATION
OFFICER	AMBULANCE STAGING
RADIO CH	LOCATION

- DATE
- TIME
- INCIDENT #
- ADDRESS
- NATURE

EQUIPMENT NEEDED AT INCIDENT

- SALVAGE COVERS
- BLANKETS
- BACKBOARDS/STRAPS
- PORTABLE OXYGEN
- BANDAGES
- IV'S
- SPLINTS/C. COLLARS
- AIRWAY SUPPLIES

OTHER:

INSTRUCTIONS FOR ARRIVING UNITS:

UNIT IDENTIFICATION	STAFF	BLS	ALS	SPECIAL EQUIPMENT	RADIO FREQ	ASSIGNMENT # 1	TIME OUT	READY	TIME OUT	ASSIGNMENT # 2	TIME OUT

APPENDIX D

COMMONWEALTH OF VIRGINIA
MASS CASUALTY INCIDENT MANAGEMENT TACTICAL WORKSHEET
PATIENT DISPOSITION TACTICAL WORKSHEET

OFFICER	*COMMAND*	
RADIO CH	LOCATION	
OFFICER	*OPERATIONS*	
RADIO CH	LOCATION	
OFFICER	*EMS/MED CONTROL*	
RADIO CH	LOCATION	
OFFICER	*TREATMENT*	
RADIO CH	LOCATION	

DATE	INCIDENT #
TIME	
ADDRESS	
NATURE	

OFFICER	*TRANSPORTATION*
RADIO CH	LOCATION
OFFICER	*TRANSPORT RECORDER*
RADIO CH	LOCATION
OFFICER	*TRANSPORT LOADER*
RADIO CH	LOCATION
OFFICER	*MEDICAL COMMUNICATIONS*
RADIO CH	LOCATION
OFFICER	*HOSPITAL COMMUNICATIONS*
RADIO CH/PHONE #	M.D.

CASUALTIES

INITIAL SURVEY APPROXIMATE # OF PATIENTS   INJURIES: MAJOR _____ MINOR _____

TRIAGE REPORT		TRANSPORT UPDATES					TOTAL TRANSPORTED
TIME							
IMMEDIATE							
DELAYED							
MINOR							
DEAD							
TOTAL							

AMBULANCE STAGING		*MEDEVAC HELICOPTER LZ*
OFFICER		OFFICER
RADIO CH LOCATION		RADIO CH LOCATION

HOSPITAL CAPACITIES

FACILITY	CAPACITY AVAILABLE			TRANSPORTED/CAPACITY USED		
	IMMEDIATE	DELAYED	MINOR	IMMEDIATE	DELAYED	MINOR

TIME OR ✓	TASKS	

MEDICAL GROUP WORKSHEET

INCIDENT NAME/LOCATION	DATE	TIME
INCIDENT COMMANDER		

MEDICAL GROUP SUPERVISOR

- TREATMENT UNIT LEADER
  - TREATMENT DISPATCH MANAGER
  - IMMEDIATE TREATMENT MANAGER
    - HOSPITAL TEAM
  - DELAYED TREATMENT MANAGER
    - HOSPITAL TEAM
  - MINOR TREATMENT MANAGER
    - HOSPITAL TEAM
- TRIAGE UNIT LEADER
  - TRIAGE PERSONNEL
  - TRANSPORTERS
  - MORGUE MANAGER
  - MEDICAL SUPPLY UNIT LEADER
- TRANSPORTATION UNIT LEADER
  - MEDICAL COMMUNICATIONS COORDINATOR
  - TRANSPORTATION RECORDER
  - AMBULANCE STAGING MANAGER

OTHER

OTHER CONSIDERATIONS	
	MEDICAL CACHES
	AIR AMBULANCE
	LAW ENFORCEMENT
	ADDITIONAL RADIO FREQUENCY(S)
	CORONER
	RED CROSS
	RELIEFS
	CHAPLAIN
	BUSES
	DEPARTMENT OF HEALTH SERVICES
	DEBRIEFING TEAMS

AMBULANCE COMPANIES

HOSPITAL TEAMS	TEAM LEADER: PHYSICIANS

COOPERATING AGENCIES

APPENDIX D

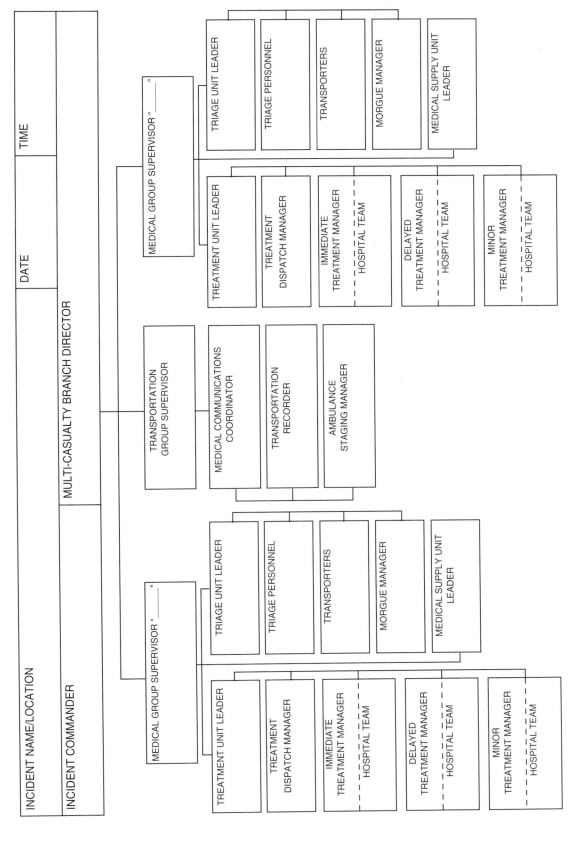

MEDICAL BRANCH WORKSHEET (PART 2)

OTHER CONSIDERATIONS

	MEDICAL CACHES	AIR AMBULANCE	LAW ENFORCEMENT	ADDITIONAL RADIO FREQUENCY(S)	CORONER	RED CROSS	RELIEFS	CHAPLAIN	BUSES	DEPARTMENT OF HEALTH SERVICES	DEBRIEFING TEAMS	

AMBULANCE COMPANIES

HOSPITAL TEAMS / TEAM LEADER PHYSICIANS

COOPERATING AGENCIES

E

Emergency Medical Incident Command Tool Box

The following sections of resource information are provided as guidelines that the Incident Commander or local jurisdiction may choose to use or adopt.

Medical Group Staffing

It is important to remember that major, disaster-level emergency medical incidents are resource intensive. The number of personnel on the scene is the critical issue, not the number of apparatus, companies, or ambulances. The example information provided in this appendix is based on a hypothetical number of patients for a given incident and is listed next to the suggested resource. For the purpose of this appendix, it is assumed that fire companies will be staffed with four members, and ambulances will have two people assigned.

NOTE: These examples of resource requirements and the staffing levels contained within them are offered as a suggested guidelines only. They may need to be adjusted based on the resources available to any particular jurisdiction.

Staffing Needs for the Extrication Unit

The general guideline for staffing the Extrication Unit is that one company (3 to 4 rescuers) for every five patients is considered reasonable. This allows immediate care to be provided when numerous patients are involved in a major incident. The goal, as resources, personnel, and priorities permit, is to provide all of the personnel and resources necessary to extricate and move patients to a designated casualty collection point, triage area, or treatment area as quickly as possible.

Staffing Needs for Initial Triage Unit Development

The following people will be needed to provide initial staffing of the Triage Unit:
- 1 Unit Leader per triage area
- 1 Morgue Manager, if required
- 1 Triage team (2 personnel) per 10 patients

- 4 Litter bearers (minimum)
- One company per 5 patients (reference to extrication/support functions)

Staffing Needs for Initial Treatment Unit Development

- 1 Unit Leader per treatment area
- 1 Immediate Care Area Manager, if needed
- 1 Delayed Care Area Manager, if needed
- 1 Minor Care Area Manager, if needed
- 1 Reassessment team or casualty collection point area (2 personnel) per 10 patients
- 1 Medical Supply Manager, as needed. This role may be initially handled by the Staging Area Manager
- 1 Treatment Dispatch Manager, as needed

Initially, one ALS fire company and one ambulance crew can establish the functions of the treatment area and then expand as needed. The types and number of treatment teams will vary and are based on the incident needs. Regardless of the size of the incident, normal span-of-control rules should be maintained. The following lists provide suggested sizing of treatment teams based on the size of the incident:

Day-to-Day, Normal to Expanded Level of Operations

Immediate Care/Red Tag: 1 ALS person, 1 BLS person per patient, and 4 litter bearers

Delayed Care/Yellow Tag: 1 BLS person per patient, 1 ALS person per 3 patients, and 4 litter bearers

Minor Care/Green Tag: 1 BLS person per 3 patients

Major Emergency Medical Incidents

Immediate Care/Red Tag: 1 ALS person, 1 BLS person per 2 patients, and 4 litter bearers

Delayed Care/Yellow Tag: 1 BLS person per 3 patients, 1 ALS person per 5 patients, and 4 litter bearers

Minor Care/Green Tag: 1 BLS person per 10 patients

Disaster Level Operations

Immediate Care/Red Tag: 1 ALS person per 3 patients, 1 BLS person per 5 patients, and 4 litter bearers

Delayed Care/Yellow Tag: 1 BLS person per 5 patients, 1 ALS person per 10 patients, and 4 litter bearers

Minor Care/Green Tag: 1 BLS person per 10 patients

Staffing Needs for Transportation Unit Development

The following people will be needed to provide initial staffing of the Transportation Unit:

- 1 Unit Leader per transport area or group supervisor, as assigned
- 1 Medical Communications Manager, as needed
- 1 Transport Recorder/Ground Ambulance Coordinator, as needed
- 1 Transport Loader (crew), as needed
- 1 Air Ambulance Coordinator and additional personnel for landing zone operations, as needed
- 1 Ambulance Staging Manager, as needed

Initially, one fire company can establish the functions of the Transportation Unit and then expand as needed.

Suggested Contents For Mass Casualty Management Kits

The contents of a mass casualty management kit should be tailored to:

- Your organization's operational concept for handling mass casualty incidents
- The number of response vehicles available
- The number of personnel available
- The manner in which your organization uses the Incident Management System

The following are suggested items that your organization may choose to include in a mass casualty management kit:

ITEM	QUANTITY:
Scene Triage and Treatment Items:	
Triage tags	Based on number carried by vehicles — suggest at least an additional 25 tags
Tarpaulins, flags, or other ways to mark patient treatment areas	1 each, RED, YELLOW, GREEN, BLACK
Triage tape kits	Based on the number carried by vehicles — suggest an additional 2 kits
Appropriate medical supplies	May be carried on vehicles as standard packs or loaded in disaster vehicles or trailers — select the method that works best for your situation — consider extra backboards, straps, splints, blankets, oxygen equipment, airway equipment, bandages, dressings, and IV sets and fluids

ITEM	QUANTITY:
Scene Control Items:	
Bullhorn	1 as minimum
Identification vests	1 each color per your procedures and marked for key staff — may include: MEDICAL GROUP, STAGING, EXTRICATION, TREATMENT, TRIAGE, TRANSPORTATION, MEDICAL COMMUNICATIONS, MORGUE, TRANSPORT RECORDER, TRANSPORT LOADER, LANDING ZONE
Area tape, traffic cones, or other markers	Several rolls to mark areas as needed according to local procedures — may be used to create movement lanes, mark vehicle staging areas, identify hazard areas
Portable lighting	As required to light treatment and management areas — may be carried as part of regular vehicle equipment or on disaster vehicles
Management Items:	
Command post flag	1 colored per your procedures
Tactical work sheets	1 large work sheet and 6 sets of standard tactical work sheets with 20 additional transportation and treatment log sheets
Clipboards	1 for each incident management system position
Ballpoint pens	1 for each clipboard plus 10 extra
Markers	1 set assorted colors for use with the large tactical work sheet
Procedures	1 copy of mass casualty standard operating procedures, current hospital patient capabilities table, and inventories of mass casualty truck/trailer units
Phone book or lists	1 set of key local emergency numbers
Maps	1 set of local road maps

Mass Casualty Incident Patient Flow

The Incident Scene

- All patients are accounted for, trapped patients are rescued/extricated.
- Patients are counted and quickly triaged.
- Triage tags are applied.
- Ambulatory patients are directed to a medically supervised area. These patients should be moved to a special part of the treatment area as soon as that area is identified.
- Nonambulatory patients are moved from the scene to a treatment area by porters.
- Patients are decontaminated (as necessary) prior to leaving the incident scene.

The Treatment Area

- Patients arriving from the incident scene are prioritized for treatment using a more in-depth assessment method (secondary triage) and triage tagged.
- Patients are placed in the treatment area and definitive/stabilizing emergency medical care is provided on the basis of triage priority.
- Separate areas are created within the treatment area for immediate, delayed, and minor care patients.
- A separate isolated area is created for patients who die in the treatment area.
- Personnel and equipment resources are allocated to patients on the basis of triage priority.
- Patients are continuously reevaluated (re-triaged).

The Transportation Area

- Hospitals are contacted to obtain information to assist with the most appropriate patient distribution to medical facilities.
- Transportation resources are assigned on the basis of triage priority.
- Patients are moved from the transportation area to the appropriate transport vehicle by litter bearers.
- Patients are transported to the most appropriate medical facility by the most appropriate means available.
- Emergency medical care and continuous reassessment is provided en route to the medical facility.

Emergency Medical Incident Categories

Multiple Victim Incidents

- Local medical resources modify field triage, treatment, and transportation procedures to handle the number of casualties.
- Local medical facilities require advanced notice to prepare for multiple patients.

Mass Casualty Incidents

Extended/Expanded Medical Incidents

- Local medical resources (including mutual aid) are available and adequate for field triage, prehospital treatment/stabilization, and transportation.
- Available local facilities are adequate and appropriate for further diagnosis and treatment.

Major Medical Incidents

- Incident produces large numbers of casualties.
- Require regional or multijurisdictional medical response for adequate mitigation.

Disasters

- Exceeds/overwhelms available regional and multijurisdictional medical resources.
- Requires assistance from state or federal sources.

Catastrophe

- Local, regional, and multijurisdictional resources concentrated toward self-survival.
- Dependent on state or federal assistance for mitigation.

F
CREDITS

The Emergency Medical Incident subcommittee brought together some of the most knowledgeable people ever assembled to produce an EMS procedures manual for the Nation's Fire Service. We are indebted to them and their department chiefs for recognizing the importance of this undertaking and for supporting their attendance at the meetings.

Chair
Tom Schwartz, Lieutenant, Fairfax County Fire and Rescue Department, Fairfax, VA

Mark Adams, Executive Director (Retired), Central Shenandoah EMS Council, Fishersville, VA

Marianne C. Anderson, Lieutenant, Anne Arundel County Fire Department, MD

Frank Borden, Assistant Chief (Retired), Los Angeles City Fire Department, CA

Rob Glover, Training Specialist, Virginia Beach Fire Department, VA

Walter Green III, Disaster Response Coordinator, Virginia Department of Health, Office of Emergency Medical Services, Richmond, VA

David Hull, Lieutenant, Ketchikan Fire Department, AK

Frank Kirk, EMS Director, Seminole County, FL

Don Lee, Captain, Los Angeles City Fire Department, CA

Paul Maniscalco, Special Operations, New York City EMS, NY

Jeffery P. Money, Battalion Chief, Brevard County, FL

Gary Morris, Deputy Chief, Phoenix Fire Department, AZ

Paul Nichols, Captain, Fairfax County Fire & Rescue Department, VA

Mike Player, Battalion Chief, York County Fire Department, VA

Bill Stevenson, EMS Director, Sussex County EMS, Georgetown, DE

Phillip Vorlander, Executive Assistant Chief, Madison Fire Department, WI